Rehabilitation and Robotics: Are They Working Well Together?

Rehabilitation and Robotics: Are They Working Well Together?

Editor

Daniele Giansanti

MDPI • Basel • Beijing • Wuhan • Barcelona • Belgrade • Manchester • Tokyo • Cluj • Tianjin

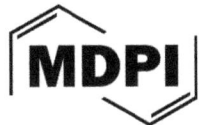

Editor
Daniele Giansanti
Centro TISP
Istituto Superiore di Sanità
Rome
Italy

Editorial Office
MDPI
St. Alban-Anlage 66
4052 Basel, Switzerland

This is a reprint of articles from the Special Issue published online in the open access journal *Healthcare* (ISSN 2227-9032) (available at: www.mdpi.com/journal/healthcare/special_issues/Robotic_Rehabilitation).

For citation purposes, cite each article independently as indicated on the article page online and as indicated below:

LastName, A.A.; LastName, B.B.; LastName, C.C. Article Title. *Journal Name* **Year**, *Volume Number*, Page Range.

ISBN 978-3-0365-4288-1 (Hbk)
ISBN 978-3-0365-4287-4 (PDF)

© 2022 by the authors. Articles in this book are Open Access and distributed under the Creative Commons Attribution (CC BY) license, which allows users to download, copy and build upon published articles, as long as the author and publisher are properly credited, which ensures maximum dissemination and a wider impact of our publications.

The book as a whole is distributed by MDPI under the terms and conditions of the Creative Commons license CC BY-NC-ND.

Contents

About the Editor vii

Preface to "Rehabilitation and Robotics: Are They Working Well Together?" ix

Daniele Giansanti
The Rehabilitation and the Robotics: Are They Going Together Well?
Reprinted from: *Healthcare* **2020**, *9*, 26, doi:10.3390/healthcare9010026 1

Daniele Giansanti
The Social Robot in Rehabilitation and Assistance: What Is the Future?
Reprinted from: *Healthcare* **2021**, *9*, 244, doi:10.3390/healthcare9030244 5

Li Liu, Yangguang Liu and Xiao-Zhi Gao
Impacts of Human Robot Proxemics on Human Concentration-Training Games with Humanoid Robots
Reprinted from: *Healthcare* **2021**, *9*, 894, doi:10.3390/healthcare9070894 15

Rossella Simeoni, Federico Colonnelli, Veronica Eutizi, Matteo Marchetti, Elena Paolini and Valentina Papalini et al.
The Social Robot and the Digital Physiotherapist: Are We Ready for the Team Play?
Reprinted from: *Healthcare* **2021**, *9*, 1454, doi:10.3390/healthcare9111454 29

Peter Bartík, Michal Vostrý, Zuzana Hudáková, Peter Šagát, Anna Lesňáková and Andrej Dukát
The Effect of Early Applied Robot-Assisted Physiotherapy on Functional Independence Measure Score in Post-Myocardial Infarction Patients
Reprinted from: *Healthcare* **2022**, *10*, 937, doi:10.3390/healthcare10050937 39

Lisa Monoscalco, Rossella Simeoni, Giovanni Maccioni and Daniele Giansanti
Information Security in Medical Robotics: A Survey on the Level of Training, Awareness and Use of the Physiotherapist
Reprinted from: *Healthcare* **2022**, *10*, 159, doi:10.3390/healthcare10010159 49

Daniele Giansanti and Rosario Alfio Gulino
The Cybersecurity and the Care Robots: A Viewpoint on the Open Problems and the Perspectives
Reprinted from: *Healthcare* **2021**, *9*, 1653, doi:10.3390/healthcare9121653 67

Giovanni Morone and Daniele Giansanti
Comment on Anwer et al. Rehabilitation of Upper Limb Motor Impairment in Stroke: A Narrative Review on the Prevalence, Risk Factors, and Economic Statistics of Stroke and State of the Art Therapies. *Healthcare* 2022, *10*, 190
Reprinted from: *Healthcare* **2022**, *10*, 846, doi:10.3390/healthcare10050846 79

Saba Anwer, Asim Waris, Syed Omer Gilani, Javaid Iqbal, Nusratnaaz Shaikh and Amit N. Pujari et al.
Reply to Morone, G.; Giansanti, D. Comment on "Anwer et al. Rehabilitation of Upper Limb Motor Impairment in Stroke: A Narrative Review on the Prevalence, Risk Factors, and Economic Statistics of Stroke and State of the Art Therapies. *Healthcare* 2022, *10*, 190"
Reprinted from: *Healthcare* **2022**, *10*, 847, doi:10.3390/healthcare10050847 83

Giovanni Morone, Antonia Pirrera, Paola Meli and Daniele Giansanti
Ethics and Automated Systems in the Health Domain: Design and Submission of a Survey on Rehabilitation and Assistance Robotics to Collect Insiders' Opinions and Perception
Reprinted from: *Healthcare* **2022**, *10*, 778, doi:10.3390/healthcare10050778 . . . . **85**

Giovanni Maccioni, Selene Ruscitto, Rosario Alfio Gulino and Daniele Giansanti
Opportunities and Problems of the Consensus Conferences in the *Care Robotics*
Reprinted from: *Healthcare* **2021**, *9*, 1624, doi:10.3390/healthcare9121624 . . . . **99**

About the Editor

Daniele Giansanti

Dr. Giansanti received: a MD in Electronic Engineering at Sapienza University, 1991, Rome. A PHD in Telecommunications and Microelectronics Engineering at Tor Vergata University, 1997, Rome. An Academic Specialization in Cognitive Psychology and Neural Networks at Sapienza University, Rome, 1997. His Academic Specialization in Medical Physics, at Sapienza University, Rome, 2005.

Dr. Giansanti was in charge of Design of VLSI Asics for DSP in the Civil Field (1991–1997) during his MD and PHD, and he served as CAE-CAD-CAM system manager and Design Engineer in the project of electronic systems (Boards and VLSI) for the Warfare at Elettronica spa (1992–2000), one of the leaders in this military field.

More importantly, he also conducts various research at ISS (the Italian NIH) (2000–today) in the following fields:

1) Biomedical Engineering and Medical Physics with the design and construction of wearable and portable devices (3 national patents).

2) Telemedicine and e-Health: technology assessment and integration of new systems in the field of the tele-rehabilitation, domiciliary monitoring, digital pathology, digital radiology.

3) Mhealth: recent interest in the field of the integration of smartphones and tablet technology in health care with particular care to the opportunities and the relevant problems of risks, abuse and regulation.

4) Acceptance and consensus in the use of robots for assistance and rehabilitation.

5) Challenges and acceptance in the use of Artificial Intelligence in Digital Radiology and Digital Pathology.

6) Cybersecurity in the health domain.

7) Technologies for frail and disable people.

He is the Professor at Sapienza and Catholic University in Rome in several courses and tutor of several theses.

He is Board Editor and reviewer in several journals. He has 126 indexed publications on Scopus and more than 200 contributes as monographies, chapters and contributes to congresses.

Preface to "Rehabilitation and Robotics: Are They Working Well Together?"

Clinical studies on the use of robotic technologies in the rehabilitation field, ranging from the field of disabling pathologies of neurological origin up to the field of injuries (included the ones into the work) and/or the support of the elderly have gained increasing attention. In the last few years, we have assisted an increasing use of the robotic devices alone and/or in association with other rehabilitation technologies. Despite the great development of robotics in the rehabilitation field, however, we are assisting to approaches differently from each other in the use and in the relevant models of care. As in other sectors, such as telemedicine, robotics is often used very limitedly to pilot and/or research projects. Just like in telemedicine, all aspects that can strengthen the use of robotics in routine clinical activities must be addressed in the international panorama with strong dedicated initiatives. There is a particular need for scholars to focus on both the innovations in this field and the problems hampering the rehabilitation robotics, to facilitate the correct and effective introduction of this technology into routine clinical programs in stable health care models. All professionals involved in rehabilitation robotics were encouraged to contribute with their experiences. This book contains contributions from various experts and different fields. Aspects of rehabilitation robotics relating to clinical experience, acceptance and emerging risks, such as cybersecurity, were addressed. Particular space was also given to ethical aspects and the related impact and to developments of social robotics and its impact in the health domain. We dedicate the book to all those involved with different roles in the rehabilitation processes of the person.

Daniele Giansanti
Editor

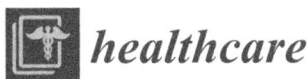 healthcare

Editorial

The Rehabilitation and the Robotics: Are They Going Together Well?

Daniele Giansanti

Centre Tisp, Istituto Superiore di Sanità, Via Regina Elena 299, 00161 Roma, Italy; daniele.giansanti@iss.it; Tel.: +39-06-49902701

Citation: Giansanti, D. The Rehabilitation and the Robotics: Are They Going Together Well? *Healthcare* **2021**, *9*, 26. https://doi.org/10.3390/healthcare9010026

Received: 25 December 2020
Accepted: 28 December 2020
Published: 30 December 2020

Publisher's Note: MDPI stays neutral with regard to jurisdictional claims in published maps and institutional affiliations.

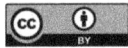

Copyright: © 2020 by the author. Licensee MDPI, Basel, Switzerland. This article is an open access article distributed under the terms and conditions of the Creative Commons Attribution (CC BY) license (https://creativecommons.org/licenses/by/4.0/).

1. Rehabilitation and the Robotics

The following problems have always existed in rehabilitation [1]:
- Operational and functional reorganization from a cerebral point of view and motor recovery seem to require therapies that require an important use of the limb associated with an innovative type of learning and/or ability with regard to new motor skills.
- Based on the previous consideration, it is evident that simple movements do not lead to maximum recovery of the rehabilitated limb.
- Based on the first consideration, it is also clear that even the use of passive exercises does not lead to optimal recovery of the affected limb.

Hence the reasoning that led to the genesis and first use of robotics as practical and effective rehabilitation tools [2,3] because they can allow administration of rehabilitation therapies that include:
1. Motivating and engaging rehabilitation exercises.
2. Training that both optimizes and maximizes the functionality of the limb.
3. An environment full of motivating stimuli.

Rehabilitation supported by the use of robotic systems can have numerous advantages [4]. In particular, it allows more intensive and tailored to the patient rehabilitation activities and services (increasing the amount and quality of therapy that can be administered) and allows all the involved actors in the team (e.g., physiotherapists, physicians, bioengineers and other figures) to set and manage some work parameters to make the rehabilitation specific and optimal for the patient (the type of exercise, the level of assistance from the robot, the force and the kinematic that the patient must exert, following the exercize).

1.1. Robotic Technological Tools Used in Rehabilitation

There are two different types of robotic technological tool (RTT) in rehabilitation for both the lower and upper limbs. The first is based on exoskeletal instruments. The second is of the end-effector type.

1.1.1. Exoskeletal-Type RTT

The exoskeletal robot, whether it is for the lower [5] or upper limbs [6], completely covers the limb, following and replicating its anthropometric characteristics and thus guiding each segment involved in the rehabilitation practice. The exoskeletons are systems with a mixture of mechanical and electronic components that constitute a mechatronic apparatus that is worn and that performs the same type of kinematic/dynamic activity practiced by the patient who wears it. These systems cover the affected limb, or at least the part of the limb affected by the clinical aspects from a rehabilitation point of view. In these systems the number of degrees of freedom is equal to that of the joints on which the rehabilitation therapy must intervene based on the objectives. Regarding the rehabilitation of the lower limbs [4] we refer to class 1 exoskeletal systems in reference to nonportable robotic systems. Class 1 belong to those nonportable robotic systems consisting of a robotic exoskeleton. In some cases there is also a body weight support (BWS) [4] type system distributed over the whole body for weight relief, a conveyor belt and a control information system including biofeedback response systems based on virtual reality. These systems are naturally used only in the clinic and partly constitute an evolution of pure BWS systems. We expressly refer to Class 2 exoskeletal systems with specific reference to portable systems that can also be used externally to the rehabilitation clinical environment.

1.1.2. End-Effector-Type RTT

In a robotic end-effector device, the input for carrying out the rehabilitation exercise comes directly from the distal part of the limb, allowing the natural kinematic activation of the movement without unnatural constraints. These systems are used for both lower [7] and upper limb [8,9] rehabilitation. The robot with the end-effector interconnects to the limb in a single point, generally a handle or a grip point for the rehabilitation of the upper limb or a pedal-like tool for the rehabilitation of the lower limbs. As regards the rehabilitation of the upper limbs with reference to end-effector systems, in some cases we speak of Cartesian systems due to some constraints that can be imposed in the trajectories also combined with specific exercises (also gamified) provided by software.

1.2. Benefits of the RTTs

Both the two RTTs produce patient benefits [4–9].

It is now well established that for the lower limbs the RTT produces various benefits, including:

- Improved trunk control.
- Improvement of the sleep-wake rhythm and reduction of perceived fatigue in carrying out daily life activities.
- Pain relief.
- Improvement in the state of mental health.
- Improvement of general anthropometric characteristics (reduction of fat mass, increase of lean mass).
- Improvement of intestinal and bladder function.

Some of these benefits are also obtained thanks to combination with specific software also based on virtual reality (VR) and/or augmented reality (AR), and also in defined protected immersive virtual environments where the rehabilitation scenarios called Cave Automatic Virtual Environment (better known with the acronym CAVE) take place.

It is now well established that for the upper limbs the use of an RTT shows several benefits, including:

- Neuromotor improvement of limb function.
- Pain relief.
- Improvement in the state of mental health
- Improvement of general anthropometric characteristics (reduction of fat mass, increase of lean mass)
- Improvement of cognitive functions.

Some of these benefits are also obtained thanks to the combination with specific software that generally offer motivating GAME and recently, in some cases, also based on virtual reality (VR) and/or augmented reality (AR).

2. New Directions to Explore and Open Problems: Aims of the Editorial

2.1. New Directions of Research and Development and First Aim of the Editorial

Currently, robotics for rehabilitation are pushing a lot of research and development and numerous new interesting directions are opening both directly connected to the robotic tools mentioned above and in support of an even wider rehabilitation process.

Some of these directions that more directly relate with motion rehabilitation [4,10,11] are:

1. To assess the effects of using robots at different phases of recovery.
2. To develop wearable robots easy and practical to wear and remove.
3. To decrease the costs also by means of new models of care.
4. To optimize and rethink the models of care based on robotics.
5. To empower the synergy and collaboration between professionals of the rehabilitation team and designers through shared and properly designed projects.
6. To make virtual reality, augmented reality, at home technologies, exoskeleton and artificial intelligence available for the treatment of cognitive and/or degenerative conditions.

Other directions, more focused to psychological support, in a wider approach to rehabilitation process are the following [12]:

1. To invest in social robots specifically designed to support during the rehabilitation phases (as for example in the care of the elderly).
2. To invest in social robots specifically designed as cultural mediators to support during communication/therapy activity (as in the care of the autism).
3. To face the problem of the empathy in robotics especially in relation to interaction with the social robots.

In light of the above, the editorial aims to stimulate scholars to report their experiences relating to various aspects of innovation on the development and use of robotics in rehabilitation both from a technological and clinical point of view. For all the above listed issues, and in particular for the 6, 7 and 8, perspective articles are welcome.

2.2. Open Problems and Second Aim of the Editorial

Despite the great development of robotics in the rehabilitation field, we are assisting to several different approaches in the use and in the relevant models of care. For example, both the rehabilitation therapies and the outcomes in the international panorama are often assessed in a different way. As in other sectors, such as telemedicine, robotics is often used very limited to pilot and/or research projects. Just like in telemedicine, all aspects that can strengthen the use of robotics in routine clinical activities must be addressed in the international panorama with strong dedicated initiatives. Through this approach, rehabilitation robotics will be able to be part of the portfolio of proposed healthcare offers in every state with a clear reimbursement of the indicated services. In light of the above, the editorial aims also to stimulate scholars to report their experiences related to these various aspects of the use of robotic technologies used in the rehabilitation centers and laboratories. From this collection obtained with heterogeneous methods, that presumably will range from the review to the mass survey, we expect to have important responses and stimuli for the international scientific community.

Conflicts of Interest: The authors declare no conflict of interest.

References

1. Bach-y-Rita, P. Late postacute neurologic rehabilitation: Neuroscience, engineering, and clinical programs. *Arch. Phys. Med. Rehabil.* **2003**, *84*, 1100–1108. [CrossRef]
2. Hidler, J.; Nichols, D.; Pelliccio, M.; Brady, K. Advances in the understanding and treatment of stroke impairment using robotic devices. *Top. Stroke Rehabil.* **2005**, *12*, 22–35. [CrossRef] [PubMed]
3. Volpe, B.T.; Huerta, P.T.; Zipse, J.L.; Rykman, A.; Edwards, D.; Dipietro, L.; Hogan, N.; Krebs, H.I. Robotic devices as therapeutic and diagnostic tools for stroke recovery. *Arch. Neurol.* **2009**, *66*, 1086–1090. [CrossRef] [PubMed]
4. Giansanti, D. *Automatized Rehabilitation of Walking and Posture: Proposals, Problems and Integration into e-Health, Rapporti ISTISAN 18/10*; Istituto Superiore di Sanità: Roma, Italy, 2019; pp. 1–50.
5. Sawicki, G.S.; Beck, O.N.; Kang, I.; Young, A.J. The exoskeleton expansion: Improving walking and running economy. *J. Neuroeng. Rehabil.* **2020**, *17*, 25. [CrossRef] [PubMed]
6. Mehrholz, J.; Pollock, A.; Pohl, M.; Kugler, J.; Elsner, B. Systematic review with network meta-analysis of randomized controlled trials of robotic-assisted arm training for improving activities of daily living and upper limb function after stroke. *J. Neuroeng. Rehabil.* **2020**, *17*, 83. [CrossRef] [PubMed]

7. Maranesi, E.; Riccardi, G.R.; Di Donna, V.; Di Rosa, M.; Fabbietti, P.; Luzi, R.; Pranno, L.; Lattanzio, F.; Bevilacqua, R. Effectiveness of Intervention Based on End- effector Gait Trainer in Older Patients with Stroke: A Systematic Review. *J. Am. Med. Dir. Assoc.* **2020**, *21*, 1036–1044. [CrossRef] [PubMed]
8. Singh, H.; Unger, J.; Zariffa, J.; Pakosh, M.; Jaglal, S.; Craven, B.C.; Musselman, K.E. Robot-assisted upper extremity rehabilitation for cervical spinal cord injuries: A systematic scoping review. *Disabil. Rehabil. Assist. Technol.* **2018**, *13*, 704–715. [CrossRef] [PubMed]
9. Molteni, F.; Gasperini, G.; Cannaviello, G.; Guanziroli, E. Exoskeleton and End-Effector Robots for Upper and Lower Limbs Rehabilitation: Narrative Review. *PM R* **2018**, *10* (Suppl. 2), S174–S188. [CrossRef] [PubMed]
10. Lennon, O.; Tonellato, M.; Del Felice, A.; Di Marco, R.; Fingleton, C.; Korik, A.; Guanziroli, E.; Molteni, F.; Guger, C.; Otner, R.; et al. A Systematic Review Establishing the Current State-of-the-Art, the Limitations, and the DESIRED Checklist in Studies of Direct Neural Interfacing with Robotic Gait Devices in Stroke Rehabilitation. *Front. Neurosci.* **2020**, *14*, 578. [CrossRef]
11. Hobbs, B.; Artemiadis, P. A Review of Robot-Assisted Lower-Limb Stroke Therapy: Unexplored Paths and Future Directions in Gait Rehabilitation. *Front. Neurorobot.* **2020**, *15*, 14–19. [CrossRef]
12. Sheridan, T.B. A review of recent research in social robotics. *Curr. Opin. Psychol.* **2020**, *36*, 7–12. [CrossRef] [PubMed]

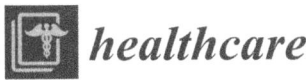 healthcare

Commentary

The Social Robot in Rehabilitation and Assistance: What Is the Future?

Daniele Giansanti

Centre Tisp, Istituto Superiore di Sanità, 00131 Rome, Italy; daniele.giansanti@iss.it; Tel.: +39-06-4990-2701

Abstract: This commentary aims to address the field of social robots both in terms of the global situation and research perspectives. It has four polarities. First, it revisits the evolutions in robotics, which, starting from collaborative robotics, has led to the diffusion of social robots. Second, it illustrates the main fields in the employment of social robots in rehabilitation and assistance in the elderly and handicapped and in further emerging sectors. Third, it takes a look at the future directions of the research development both in terms of clinical and technological aspects. Fourth, it discusses the opportunities and limits, starting from the development and clinical use of social robots during the COVID-19 pandemic to the increase of ethical discussion on their use.

Keywords: e-health; medical devices; m-health; rehabilitation; robotics; organization models; artificial intelligence; electronic surveys; social robots; collaborative robots

Citation: Giansanti, D. The Social Robot in Rehabilitation and Assistance: What Is the Future?. *Healthcare* **2021**, *9*, 244. https://doi.org/10.3390/healthcare9030244

Academic Editor: Tin-Chih Toly Chen

Received: 21 January 2021
Accepted: 14 February 2021
Published: 25 February 2021

Publisher's Note: MDPI stays neutral with regard to jurisdictional claims in published maps and institutional affiliations.

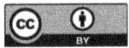

Copyright: © 2021 by the author. Licensee MDPI, Basel, Switzerland. This article is an open access article distributed under the terms and conditions of the Creative Commons Attribution (CC BY) license (https://creativecommons.org/licenses/by/4.0/).

1. Introduction

We can certainly place among the most marvelous and shocking technological developments of recent years those of collaborative robotics and, among them, those related to social robotics.

The social robot represents an important technological issue to deeply explore both from a technological and clinical point of view. It has been highlighted in an editorial in the Special Issue of the journal Healthcare entitled "Rehabilitation and Robotics: Are They Working Well Together?" [1]. Among the most important directions in the development of social robotics connected to assistance and rehabilitation we find, in a wider approach to the process of rehabilitation and assistance, the following:

- To invest in social robots specifically designed as support during rehabilitation phases (such as, for example, in the care of the elderly).
- To invest in social robots specifically designed as cultural mediators to support during communication/therapy activity (such as in the care of autism).
- To address the problem of empathy in robotics, especially in relation to interaction with social robots.

In fact, starting from the experiences of collaborative robotics, social robots have spread and are opening new opportunities in the field of the rehabilitation and assistance of fragile subjects with different types of problems, ranging from neuromotor disabilities to those of a communicative and psychological type. A particular acceleration in this area has also certainly been due to the COVID-19 pandemic. The need to maintain social distancing, combined with that of (a) ensuring the continuity of care and (b) giving a communicative type of support, has prompted us to look in the direction of social robots as a possible solution at hand: a real lifebuoy. We have, therefore, increasingly begun to look at social robots both, in a more futuristic way, as a potential substitute for human health care and rehabilitation and, in a more realistic and ethically acceptable way, as a reliable possible mediator/facilitator between humans in the field of rehabilitation and assistance. To tell the truth, even before the pandemic, some of the "social" potential of robots had begun to scare us. Recent challenges in some games (which involve a high degree of social interactions based on tactics) between robots and humans have in fact shown us how the computational abilities of robots have definitively knocked out what we previously believed to be the primacy of human intelligence. In 2016, years after Deep Blue's [2–4] famous defeat of Kasparov at chess [5,6], a computer called AlphaGo [7] beat the world champion of *Go* [8,9], a game much more complex than chess; in fact, in this game, the possible options for the first move are 361 (20 in chess) and the second are 130,000 (400 in chess!). According to the scholars of this game, to win, it is necessary to be familiar with the models of social interaction that go far beyond simple computation! The following questions immediately emerge:

- With AlphaGo, are we crossing the threshold between the two forms of artificial and human intelligence, and what does this entail for future developments?
- What is the boundary between a social robot and a powerful computer?
- Does a social robot have at least a mechatronic body (AlphaGo does not have one)?
- Is an interactive video connected to a computer attached to a mobile body/column sufficient to characterize a social robot?
- What degree of autonomy must a social robot have in any case?
- Is all of this ethically acceptable?

As scholars in the field of assistance and rehabilitation, we also question ourselves on these points, which touch on important aspects of (a) scientific research in mechatronics, neuroscience, artificial intelligence and bioengineering; (b) bioethics; and (c) economics and politics, ranging from regulatory to organizational aspects. In light of this, taking into account the focus of this Special Issue, the goal of our study is mainly to produce a commentary that is useful in the field of research without, however, where possible, neglecting the other aspects. In particular, we wish to highlight in this study a map point and a conceptual contextualization of these technologies starting from the roots, which are based on corobotics, and understand what direction these devices are taking and what we can expect in the future.

2. The Social Robot as an Evolution of the Collaborative Robot

2.1. Collaborative Robots

The term *corobot* or *cobot* derives from the merging of the term collaborative with the term robot [10]. It appeared in the Wall Street Journal in its millennium edition on 1 January 2000 [11] and refers to technologies used since 1996 thanks to the ingenuity of two professors from Northwestern University, J. Edward Colgate and Michael Peshkin. Cobots are robots designed to interact with humans from a certain work environment and in an interaction workspace. Currently, among the robotics sectors, this sector represents one of the greatest developments.

The International Federation of Robotics [12], a professional, nonprofit organization, recognizes two types of robots: industrial robots used in automation and collaborative robots that can be of service for professional and home use. In the field of collaborative robots, there are four groupings:

1. Reactive collaboration: the robot responds to the movement of the worker in real time;
2. Cooperation: the human and robot are both in motion and work simultaneously;
3. Sequential collaboration: the human and robot share part or all of a workspace but do not work simultaneously;
4. Coexistence: there is no shared workspace, but the human and robot work together.

2.2. Social Robots

The ability to interact and work with humans is a characteristic of collaborative robots. However, if this interaction and work activity is more characterized by social interaction until it becomes the key role, then we are dealing with a social robot, also called a socially interactive robot [13].

In other words, social robots are collaborative robots evolved/specialized in social interaction, and their work is social interaction.

We must take into account that robots are and will be increasingly part of our lives. Interaction with artificial intelligence in workplaces, shops, healthcare facilities and numerous other meeting places will be increasingly frequent.

Social robots (SRs) in their collaborative interaction are capable [13] of:

- Establishing and maintaining social relationships;
- Learning social skills development and role models;
- Using "natural" signals, such as gestures and gaze;
- Expressing emotions and are able to perceive them;
- Communicating with high-level dialog;
- Expressing one's own personality and distinctive character.

SRs can be used for a variety of purposes; for example, as educational tools and therapeutic aids. There are several examples of SRs designed for use by elderly people [14–17], in nursing homes or in hospitals, for example, to:

(a) Support certain motor activities;
(b) Support the elderly during feeding;
(c) Support them in drug therapy; for example, by reminding them to take a drug;
(d) Support them from a cognitive point of view; for example, by stimulating them with games and supporting them from the point of view of communicative interaction, even as simple company;
(e) Or, more generally, provide support as a hospital assistant.

For this reason, SRs are being considered among the key gerontechnologies [17] for the future.

In the COVID-19 era, there has been an increase in the use of SRs in the above-listed desirable activities due to the necessary supervening obligation of social distancing to combat the pandemic [18]. One nonexhaustive example of this is the use of Pepper [7,19] in the UK in this field during the COVID-19 pandemic [20]. Social robotics can also be useful as:

(f) Support in the rehabilitation therapy of communication disabilities such as autism or others, where the robot can represent a useful tool full of stimuli for children [18,21–28].

However, the robots can also be used in the home environment while integrated with home automation technologies by supporting the activities listed above in the elderly. Wakamaru [29], for example, can be integrated into domotics with a wide range of support possibilities. Additionally, so-called home-telepresence robots are headed in this direction. They act as home management mediators/facilitators, allowing communication with other people by means of proper devices (cameras, speakers, microphones, etc.) and improving the subject's safety. Kuri [30] and JIBO [31] are a family of robots that includes telepresence.

3. Research Directions in Social Robots

3.1. A Possible Categorization as a Reference

In an interesting review, Sheridan [32] recently categorized the research direction in the field of SRs as follows: (1) Affect, Personality and Adaptation; (2) Sensing and Control for Action; (3) Assistance to the Elderly and Handicapped; (4) Toys and Markets. We summarize this briefly, referring to the review for an in-depth view.

3.1.1. Affect, Personality and Adaptation

The research in this direction [32–38] concerns using information about the user in order to adapt the SRs to the user's particular needs and performance intentions, thereby improving acceptance; therefore several studies focus, for example, on how movements of the robot's body parts imitate human emotions to express different emotions such as anger, disgust, fear, happiness, sadness and surprise.

3.1.2. Sensing and Control for Action

This section considers research that focuses more on the physical interaction between humans and SRs, with consideration to bioengineering solutions [32,39–65]. While safety is essential to human–robot collaboration for industrial manipulation and carefully avoiding collisions, in SRs, the guard is different, and great attention is given to the social tasks, such as applying makeup to the human face. More attention has been given to the problem of motion planning, not only for collision avoidance (obviously, safety remains a basic aspect to consider) but also for human likeness. The touch of a robot, in many cases, for example, induces a positive response in a human, so this aspect must be carefully considered.

3.1.3. Assistance to the Elderly and Handicapped

This is one social robot application that has received much attention [32,66–76]. For example, families coping with a relative with autism often struggle with social and emotional communication. In the case of the elderly, the research directions confirm what has been discussed above in Section 1. In the case of the research on the use of robots for children with autism, some gaps have been identified and reported by Sheridan [32], such as diversity in focus, bias in the research toward specific behavior impairments, the effectiveness of the human–robot interaction after impairment and the use of robot-based motor rehabilitation in autism.

3.1.4. Toys and the Market for Social Robots in General

Here, Sheridan [23] makes the important consideration that for user acceptance, government regulator acceptance and sales appeal, engineering/research related to social psychological and human factors should be applied to social robots. This is especially true for children's toys because children are the most vulnerable of the various user categories. It should be considered that most of the sales of social robots today are for children's toys as it is possible to see over the web.

3.2. Further Personal Considerations

I agree with the categorization identified by Sheridan [32], and I believe that it can be used as a reference for evaluating the future developments of social robots, with particular reference to the assistance and rehabilitation sectors. Without introducing new categorizations and focusing on the rehabilitation sector, I believe that two recent, further considerations are worthy of note. The first is the introduction of a sort of robot-based pet therapy through robots with the appearance of animals. The second is the impact of the research and clinical applications on SRs, as partly anticipated in Section 2 due to the COVID-19 pandemic. Both topics are translational with respect to the four categories described above.

3.2.1. Social-Animal-Like Robot for Pet Therapy

The pet therapy is identified as a complementary intervention that strengthens traditional treatments and can be used on patients suffering from various pathologies, with the aim to improve their state of health, thanks to the human–animal interaction. It has been proved that the presence of an animal (e.g., dog, cat, rubbit) improves both the emotional relationship and the work with the patient, favoring the interaction, attention and in general the communication channel and stimulating the active participation of the subject. Pet therapy is often used in dedicated interventions.

Pet therapy is now finding fertile ground in SRs. Two examples of this are the two social-animal-like-robots Paro and Robear. Paro was designed by Takanori Shibata in early 1993 [77]. It was designed on the basis of a puppy seal. Paro features a complex mechatronic, with tactile sensors covering its fur, touch-sensitive whiskers and actuators that quietly move its limbs and body.

Thanks to this design, it responds to cuddles by moving its tail and opening and closing its eyes, memorizes faces, follows the guard and learns actions, generating positive reactions. Among the principal applications [15,16], it is possible to find the same applications of pet therapy in (a) reducing psychological disorders such as anxiety and depression and (b) improving communication skills and (c) the levels of attention and participation. Therefore, the social robot Paro also acts as a rehabilitation therapist. It has been used in rehabilitation therapies on the elderly (for example, with dementia) and on children with autism. Paro is a social companion for those who interact with him, encouraging effects such as increased participation, increased levels of attention and new social performances, such as cooperative attention and interaction [15,16,78–85]. Robear [86] is a white, bear-shaped robot that lifts and helps patients in wheelchairs to move to bed or go to the bathroom. It is a special robot nurse made by the Riken Brain Science Institute [87] that is conquering hospitals in Japan for its efficiency and "sweetness." Robear is driven by software and three different types of sensors, including "tactile" structures made of rubber. Weighing approximately 140 kg, Robear is strong and agile enough to (a) gently lift the patient from the bed to the wheelchair, (b) help them stand up and (c) move quickly. While the first example, represented by Paro, is a clear example of a pure robot-based pet therapy, the second, Robear, is an example of the application of both robot-based pet therapy and robot-based caregiving, which could also contribute to avoiding caregiver burning during the complex activities of assistance, especially during the COVID-19 pandemic. It should also be considered that many fragile subjects prefer more to be manipulated by a social robot (Robear in this case) than a human caregiver.

3.2.2. Social Robots and COVID-19

The COVID-19 pandemic has dramatically brought to the fore the problem of the frailty of the elderly. Often the elderly were subjected to forced isolation to avoid contagion. This has resulted in both difficulties in health care (including psychological) and the appearance of disturbing factors such as fear, anxiety and other psychological disorders. Their functional capabilities also generally declined during this period.

To try to minimize the problem, some nursing homes have started using robots to take care of the elderly to try to alleviate their loneliness while supporting them from a mental health point of view. An example of this, as briefly anticipated in Section 2, is the use of Pepper [17] in the UK. SRs, including the previously reported Robear [86], have provided an impetus in research and clinical application during the COVID-19 pandemic. At the end of the pandemic, it will be possible to completely assess this and make a map point.

4. Conclusions

The last evolution of collaborative robots (historically proposed for collaboration with human subjects) [10] is the capability to play the role of an interactive social communicator and, therefore, to be a social robot [13]. This new role is showing high potential in both the direction of rehabilitation and assistance of subjects with disabilities, especially the fragile and handicapped. SRs have particularly demonstrated potential both in the care of the elderly and children with communication disabilities, such as autism [9–22]. Recently, we have also witnessed boosted activity both in the research and clinical applications of SRs caused by the COVID-19 pandemic. In fact, SRs present a chance to allow the continuity of care and communication and psychological support in situations where there are rules/initiatives to maintain social distancing to avoid infection; in other terms, a kind of lifebuoy [17,18]. The research direction in the field of SRs has been clearly detected. In an interesting review, Sheridan [32] recently categorized the research direction in this field of SRs as follows: (1) Affect, Personality and Adaptation; (2) Sensing and Control for Action; (3) Assistance to the Elderly and Handicapped; (4) Toys and Markets. As transversal fields of this research direction, I have detected the clear introduction of robot-based pet therapy [15,16,78–86] and the impact of the COVID-19 pandemic on the research activity [17,18]. The latter opened much discussion around the use of SRs in rehabilitation and assistance, complimenting the economic and ethical sphere. Ethical issues have arisen around the key question that SRs cannot provide true selflessness, compassion and warmth, which should be at the heart of an assistance system. Scholars of epistemology are worried that SRs, with increased use, could even increase long-term loneliness, reducing the actual contact people have with humans and increasing a sense of disconnection. This, obviously, is not applicable when SRs are used either as facilitators or mediators among humans, as in most cases in domotics or in some applications in the care of autism, such as the robot Kaspar [88–91].

It is precisely this role that makes us reflect on the further opportunities of SRs in telerehabilitation applications that can occur in three important sectors:

- As facilitators/mediators to put fragile and/or needy subjects in contact with the health system and/or family members for more complete support of rehabilitation monitoring.
- As support in a more tailored patient-centered therapy by adapting SRs to the patient's telerehabilitation needs.
- In the domiciliation of care also integrated on the basis of the previous point, with the emerging robotic rehabilitation technologies of the upper and lower limbs integrated into the telerehabilitative pathways and processes.

When we reflect on SRs, and if we are worried about the above-listed problems (increasing loneliness, reducing contacts, etc.), we must also see the flip side of the coin; that is to say that, in this pandemic season, a robot of this type could provide answers to many problems that are encountered in nursing homes and hospitals, such as lack of personnel. In times of lockdown, many elderly and disabled people are left completely alone in their homes and sometimes without adequate health care. Furthermore, even leaving out the COVID-19 pandemic, there was already a problem of assistance (worldwide and in every period) for the elderly, the frail, the disabled, the sick, the lonely and the non self-sufficient. My opinion is that, in general, robotic caregivers should not only be viewed with suspicion but also as a possible opportunity for support. There is no doubt that robotics will be an important part of the health and care of the future. The robots will assist in surgical interventions (in presence or remotely), rehabilitation, in home automation, they will take care of hospital hygiene, dispense lunch and medicines and support of various kinds in general. It is certainly true that robots are not currently able to express the emotions of a human being, however they can do a job in a precise and effective way and could be of great help in dealing with the problems of disability and many problems in health care.

From an economic point of view, it is very interesting for insurance companies under various aspects, ranging from the possibility of developing new insurance formulas that revolve around the use of care-robots, as well as the introduction of new policies that cover the risks of using robots. As for other applications of artificial intelligence, a key point for the diffusion of SRs will clearly be the opinion and the acceptance, the so-called last yard, of all the involved actors, ranging from physicians, nurses and caregivers to patients with their familiars. Therefore, it will be necessary to set up dedicated studies based on dedicated large surveys [92,93] to face the last yard, in which artificial intelligence cannot fail to play a key role [94], given that artificial intelligence will be, for example, fundamental for specifying the level and characteristics of the empathy of social robots in the near future. All this is of basic importance because, according to studies focused on bibliometric indicators, we are witnessing significant growth in this sector. In the study reported in [95], for example, it is documented that the field started growing since the mid-1990s, and after 2006 [95], we can observe a larger amount of publications. The authors [95] obtained academic article data from the robotics and the social robotics fields, highlighting the important increasing number of publications on SRs (a) by number of articles and (b) proportion in relation to all-robotics research. Furthermore, now, official studies show that the social robots market is (https://www.mordorintelligence.com/industry-reports/social_robots_market) [96] estimated to grow at a compound annual growth rate of about 14% over the forecast period 2021 to 2026 thanks to the rise of research in the field of artificial intelligence (AI), natural language processing (NLP) and the development of platforms such as the robotic operating system, which enabled the rise of social robotics.

Funding: This research received no external funding.

Conflicts of Interest: The author declares no conflict of interest.

References

1. Giansanti, D. The Rehabilitation and the Robotics: Are They Going Together Well? *Health* **2020**, *9*, 26. [CrossRef] [PubMed]
2. Heßler, M. Der Erfolg der "Dummheit". *NTM Z. Gesch. Wiss. Tech. Med.* **2017**, *25*, 1–33. [CrossRef] [PubMed]
3. Sverzellati, N.; Brillet, P.-Y. When Deep Blue first defeated Kasparov: Is a machine stronger than a radiologist at predicting prognosis in idiopathic pulmonary fibrosis? *Eur. Respir. J.* **2017**, *49*, 1602144. [CrossRef]
4. Kasparov, G. Strategic intensity: A conversation with world chess champion Garry Kasparov. *Harv. Bus. Rev.* **2005**, *83*, 49–53. [PubMed]
5. Deep Blue. Available online: https://www.sciencedirect.com/science/article/pii/S0004370201001291 (accessed on 22 February 2021).
6. Deep Blue Defeats Garry Kasparov in Chess Match. Available online: https://www.history.com/this-day-in-history/deep-blue-defeats-garry-kasparov-in-chess-match (accessed on 22 February 2021).
7. Kim, H. AI, Big Data, and Robots for the Evolution of Biotechnology. *Genom. Inform.* **2019**, *17*, e44. [CrossRef] [PubMed]
8. AlphaGo. Available online: https://deepmind.com/research/case-studies/alphago-the-story-so-far (accessed on 22 February 2021).
9. The Evolution of Computing: AlphaGo. Available online: https://ieeexplore.ieee.org/document/7499782 (accessed on 22 February 2021).
10. Matthews, P.; Greenspan, S. *Automation and Collaborative Robotics: A Guide to the Future of Work*; Apress: New York, NY, USA, 2020.
11. 20 Years Later: Cobots Co-Opt Assembly Lines. Available online: https://www.mccormick.northwestern.edu/news/articles/2016/08/twenty-years-later-cobots-co-opt-assembly-lines.html (accessed on 22 February 2021).
12. International Federation of Robotics. Available online: https://ifr.org/ (accessed on 22 February 2021).
13. Korn, O. *Social Robots: Technological, Societal and Ethical Aspects of Human-Robot Interaction*; Springer: Berlin/Heidelberg, Germany, 2019.
14. Ziaeetabar, F.; Pomp, J.; Pfeiffer, S.; El-Sourani, N.; Schubotz, R.I.; Tamosiunaite, M.; Wörgötter, F. Using enriched semantic event chains to model human action prediction based on (minimal) spatial information. *PLoS ONE* **2020**, *15*, e0243829. [CrossRef]
15. Hirt, J.; Ballhausen, N.; Hering, A.; Kliegel, M.; Beer, T.; Meyer, G. Social Robot Interventions for People with Dementia: A Systematic Review on Effects and Quality of Reporting. *J. Alzheimer's Dis.* **2021**, *79*, 773–792. [CrossRef]
16. Pu, L.; Moyle, W.; Jones, C.; Todorovic, M. The effect of a social robot intervention on sleep and motor activity of people living with dementia and chronic pain: A pilot randomized controlled trial. *Maturitas* **2021**, *144*, 16–22. [CrossRef]
17. Chen, K. Use of Gerontechnology to Assist Older Adults to Cope with the COVID-19 Pandemic. *J. Am. Med. Dir. Assoc.* **2020**, *21*, 983–984. [CrossRef] [PubMed]
18. Ghiță, A.Ș.; Gavril, A.F.; Nan, M.; Hoteit, B.; Awada, I.A.; Sorici, A.; Mocanu, I.G.; Florea, A.M. The AMIRO Social Robotics Framework: Deployment and Evaluation on the Pepper Robot. *Sensors* **2020**, *20*, 7271. [CrossRef]
19. Pepper. Available online: https://robots.ieee.org/robots/pepper/ (accessed on 22 February 2021).
20. Robots to be Introduced in UK Care Homes to Allay Loneliness—That's Inhuman. Available online: https://theconversation.com/robots-to-be-introduced-in-uk-care-homes-to-allay-loneliness-thats-inhuman-145879 (accessed on 22 February 2021).
21. Naffa, H.; Fain, M. Performance measurement of ESG-themed megatrend investments in global equity markets using pure factor portfolios methodology. *PLoS ONE* **2020**, *15*, e0244225. [CrossRef] [PubMed]
22. Lewis, T.T.; Kim, H.; Darcy-Mahoney, A.; Waldron, M.; Lee, W.H.; Park, C.H. Robotic uses in pediatric care: A comprehensive review. *J. Pediatr. Nurs.* **2021**, *58*, 65–75. [CrossRef] [PubMed]
23. Soares, E.E.; Bausback, K.; Beard, C.L.; Higinbotham, M.; Bunge, E.L.; Gengoux, G.W. Social Skills Training for Autism Spectrum Disorder: A Meta-analysis of In-person and Technological Interventions. *J. Technol. Behav. Sci.* **2020**, 1–15. [CrossRef]
24. Egido-García, V.; Estévez, D.; Corrales-Paredes, A.; Terrón-López, M.-J.; Velasco-Quintana, P.-J. Integration of a Social Robot in a Pedagogical and Logopedic Intervention with Children: A Case Study. *Sensors* **2020**, *20*, 6483. [CrossRef] [PubMed]
25. So, W.-C.; Cheng, C.-H.; Law, W.-W.; Wong, T.; Lee, C.; Kwok, F.-Y.; Lee, S.-H.; Lam, K.-Y. Robot dramas may improve joint attention of Chinese-speaking low-functioning children with autism: Stepped wedge trials. *Disabil. Rehabil. Assist. Technol.* **2020**, 1–10. [CrossRef]
26. Sandgreen, H.; Frederiksen, L.H.; Bilenberg, N. Digital Interventions for Autism Spectrum Disorder: A Meta-analysis. *J. Autism Dev. Disord.* **2020**, 1–15. [CrossRef]
27. Pontikas, C.-M.; Tsoukalas, E.; Serdari, A. A map of assistive technology educative instruments in neurodevelopmental disorders. *Disabil. Rehabil. Assist. Technol.* **2020**, *30*, 1–9. [CrossRef]
28. Jain, S.; Thiagarajan, B.; Shi, Z.; Clabaugh, C.; Matarić, M.J. Modeling engagement in long-term, in-home socially assistive robot interventions for children with autism spectrum disorders. *Sci. Robot.* **2020**, *5*, eaaz3791. [CrossRef]

29. Wakamaru. Available online: https://robots.ieee.org/robots/wakamaru/ (accessed on 22 February 2021).
30. Kuri. Available online: https://robots.ieee.org/robots/kuri/ (accessed on 22 February 2021).
31. Jibo. Available online: https://robots.ieee.org/robots/jibo/ (accessed on 22 February 2021).
32. Sheridan, T.B. A review of recent research in social robotics. *Curr. Opin. Psychol.* **2020**, *36*, 7–12. [CrossRef] [PubMed]
33. Cerasa, A.; Ruta, L.; Marino, F.; Biamonti, G.; Pioggia, G. Brief Report: Neuroimaging Endophenotypes of Social Robotic Applications in Autism Spectrum Disorder. *J. Autism Dev. Disord.* **2020**, 1–5. [CrossRef]
34. Martins, G.S.; Santos, L.; Dias, J. User-Adaptive Interaction in Social Robots: A Survey Focusing on Non-physical Interaction. *Int. J. Soc. Robot.* **2018**, *11*, 185–205. [CrossRef]
35. Johnson, D.O.; Cuijpers, R.H. Investigating the Effect of a Humanoid Robot's Head Position on Imitating Human Emotions. *Int. J. Soc. Robot.* **2018**, *11*, 65–74. [CrossRef]
36. Willemse, C.J.A.M.; van Erp, J.B.F. Social touch in human–robot interaction: Robot-initiated touches can induce positive responses without extensive prior bonding. *Int. J. Soc. Robot.* **2019**, *11*, 285–304. [CrossRef]
37. Block, A.E.; Kuchenbecker, K.J. Softness, Warmth, and Responsiveness Improve Robot Hugs. *Int. J. Soc. Robot.* **2018**, *11*, 49–64. [CrossRef]
38. Palanica, A.; Thommandram, A.; Fossat, Y. Adult Verbal Comprehension Performance is Better from Human Speakers than Social Robots, but only for Easy Questions. *Int. J. Soc. Robot.* **2019**, *11*, 359–369. [CrossRef]
39. Ruijten, P.A.M.; Haans, A.; Ham, J.; Midden, C.J.H. Perceived Human-Likeness of Social Robots: Testing the Rasch Model as a Method for Measuring Anthropomorphism. *Int. J. Soc. Robot.* **2019**, *11*, 477–494. [CrossRef]
40. Lupowski, P.; Rybka, M.; Dziedic, D.; Wlodarczyk, W. The background context condition for the uncanny valley hypothesis. *Int. J. Soc. Robot.* **2019**, *11*, 25–33. [CrossRef]
41. Hoorn, J.F.; Konijn, E.A.; Pontier, M.A. Dating a synthetic character is like dating a man. *Int. J. Soc. Robot.* **2019**, *11*, 235–253. [CrossRef]
42. Bruno, B.; Recchiuto, C.T.; Papadopoulos, I.; Saffiotti, A.; Koulouglioti, C.; Menicatti, R.; Mastrogiovanni, F.; Zaccaria, R.; Sgorbissa, A. Knowledge Representation for Culturally Competent Personal Robots: Requirements, Design Principles, Implementation, and Assessment. *Int. J. Soc. Robot.* **2019**, *11*, 515–538. [CrossRef]
43. Carlson, Z.; Lemmon, L.; Higgins, M.; Frank, D.; Shahrezaie, R.S.; Feil-Seifer, D. Perceived Mistreatment and Emotional Capability Following Aggressive Treatment of Robots and Computers. *Int. J. Soc. Robot.* **2019**, *11*, 727–739. [CrossRef]
44. Stroessner, S.J.; Benitez, J. The social perception of humanoid and non-humanaoid robots: Effects of gendered and machinelike features. *Int. J. Soc. Robot.* **2019**, *11*, 305–315. [CrossRef]
45. Wang, B.; Rau, P.-L.P. Influence of Embodiment and Substrate of Social Robots on Users' Decision-Making and Attitude. *Int. J. Soc. Robot.* **2018**, *11*, 411–421. [CrossRef]
46. Shariati, A.; Shahab, M.; Meghdari, A.; Nobaveh, A.A.; Rafatnejad, R.; Mozafari, B. Virtual Reality Social Robot Platform: A Case Study on Arash Social Robot. In Proceedings of the International Conference on Social Robotics 2018, Qingdao, China, 28–30 November 2018; Springer International Publishing: Berlin/Heidelberg, Germany, 2018; pp. 551–560.
47. De Graaf, M.M.A.; Allouch, S.B. Exploring influencing for the acceptance of social robots. *Robot. Auton. Syst.* **2013**, *61*, 1476–1486. [CrossRef]
48. Homma, Y.; Suzuki, K. A Robotic Brush with Surface Tracing Motion Applied to the Face. *Lect. Notes Comput. Sci.* **2018**, *2018*, 513–522. [CrossRef]
49. Turnwald, A.; Wollherr, D. Human-Like Motion Planning Based on Game Theoretic Decision Making. *Int. J. Soc. Robot.* **2019**, *11*, 151–170. [CrossRef]
50. Erlich, S.K.; Cheng, G. A feasibility study for validating robot actions using EEG-based error-related potentials. *Int. J. Soc. Robot.* **2019**, *11*, 271–283. [CrossRef]
51. Heimerdinger, M.; Laviers, A. Modeling the Interactions of Context and Style on Affect in Motion Perception: Stylized Gaits Across Multiple Environmental Contexts. *Int. J. Soc. Robot.* **2019**, *11*, 495–513. [CrossRef]
52. Kaushik, R.; Laviers, A. Imitating Human Movement Using a Measure of Verticality to Animate Low Degree-of-Freedom Non-humanoid Virtual Characters. In Proceedings of the International Conference on Social Robotics 2018, Qingdao, China, 28–30 November 2018; Springer International Publishing: Berlin/Heidelberg, Germany, 2018; pp. 588–598.
53. Hamandi, M.; Hatay, E.; Fazli, P. Predicting the Target in Human-Robot Manipulation Tasks. In Proceedings of the International Conference on Social Robotics 2018, Qingdao, China, 28–30 November 2018; Springer International Publishing: Berlin/Heidelberg, Germany, 2018; pp. 580–587.
54. Papenmeier, F.; Uhrig, M.; Kirsch, A. Human Understanding of Robot Motion: The Role of Velocity and Orientation. *Int. J. Soc. Robot.* **2018**, *11*, 75–88. [CrossRef]
55. Liu, T.; Wang, J.; Hutchinson, S.; Meng, M.Q.-H. Skeleton-Based Human Action Recognition by Pose Specificity and Weighted Voting. *Int. J. Soc. Robot.* **2018**, *11*, 219–234. [CrossRef]
56. Kostavelis, I.; Vasileiadis, E.; Skartados, E.; Kargakos, A.; Giakoumis, D.; Bouganis, C.S.; Tzovaris, D. Understanding of human behaviorwith a robotic agent through daily activity analysis. *Int. J. Soc. Robot.* **2019**, *11*, 437–462. [CrossRef]
57. Kaushik, R.; Laviers, A. Imitation of Human Motion by Low Degree-of-Freedom Simulated Robots and Human Preference for Mappings Driven by Spinal, Arm, and Leg Activity. *Int. J. Soc. Robot.* **2019**, *11*, 765–782. [CrossRef]

58. Sprute, D.; Tönnies, K.; König, M. A Study on Different User Interfaces for Teaching Virtual Borders to Mobile Robots. *Int. J. Soc. Robot.* **2018**, *11*, 373–388. [CrossRef]
59. Radmard, S.; Moon, A.; Croft, E.A. Impacts of Visual Occlusion and Its Resolution in Robot-Mediated Social Collaborations. *Int. J. Soc. Robot.* **2018**, *11*, 105–121. [CrossRef]
60. Yoon, H.S.; Jang, J.; Kim, J. Multi-pose face recognition method for social robot. In Proceedings of the International Conference on Social Robotics 2018, Qingdao, China, 28–30 November 2018; pp. 609–619.
61. Karatas, N.; Tamura, S.; Fushiki, M.; Okada, M. The Effects of Driving Agent Gaze Following Behaviors on Human-Autonomous Car Interaction. In Proceedings of the International Conference on Social Robotics 2018, Qingdao, China, 28–30 November 2018; Springer International Publishing: Berlin/Heidelberg, Germany, 2018; pp. 541–550.
62. Li, H.; Yihun, Y.; He, H. MagicHand: In-Hand Perception of Object Characteristics for Dexterous Manipulation. In Proceedings of the International Conference on Social Robotics 2018, Qingdao, China, 28–30 November 2018; Springer International Publishing: Berlin/Heidelberg, Germany, 2018; pp. 523–532.
63. Yamashita, Y.; Ishihara, H.; Ikeda, T.; Asada, M. Investigation of Causal Relationship Between Touch Sensations of Robots and Personality Impressions by Path Analysis. *Int. J. Soc. Robot.* **2018**, *11*, 141–150. [CrossRef]
64. Spatola, N.; Belletier, C.; Chausse, P.; Augustinova, M.; Normand, A.; Barra, V.; Ferrand, L.; Huguet, P. Improved Cognitive Control in Presence of Anthropomorphized Robots. *Int. J. Soc. Robot.* **2019**, *11*, 463–476. [CrossRef]
65. Komatsubara, T.; Shiomi, M.; Kaczmarek, T.; Kanda, T.; Ishiguro, H. Estimating Children's Social Status Through Their Interaction Activities in Classrooms with a Social Robot. *Int. J. Soc. Robot.* **2019**, *11*, 35–48. [CrossRef]
66. Ismail, L.I.; Verhoeven, T.; Dambre, J.; Wyffels, F. Leveraging robotics reseach for children with autism: A review. *Int. J. Soc. Robot.* **2019**, *11*, 389–410. [CrossRef]
67. Jonaiti, M.; Henaff, P. Robot-based motor rehabilitation in autism: A systematic review. In Proceedings of the International Conference on Social Robotics 2018, Qingdao, China, 28–30 November 2018; pp. 1–12.
68. Alhaddad, A.Y.; Cabibihan, J.-J.; Bonarini, A. Head Impact Severity Measures for Small Social Robots Thrown During Meltdown in Autism. *Int. J. Soc. Robot.* **2018**, *11*, 255–270. [CrossRef]
69. Yoshikawa, Y.; Kumazake, H.; Matsumoto, Y.; Miyao, M.; Ishiguru, H.; Shimaya, J. Communication support vis a tele-operated robot for easier talking: Case/laboratory study of individuals with/ without autism spectrum disorder. *Int. J. Soc. Robot.* **2019**, *11*, 171–184.
70. Parviainen, J.; Turja, T.; Van Aerschot, L. Robots and Human Touch in Care: Desirable and Non-desirable Robot Assistance. In Proceedings of the International Conference on Social Robotics 2018, Qingdao, China, 28–30 November 2018; Springer International Publishing: Berlin/Heidelberg, Germany, 2018; pp. 533–540.
71. Karunarathne, D.; Morales, Y.; Nomura, T.; Kanda, T.; Ishiguro, H. Will Older Adults Accept a Humanoid Robot as a Walking Partner? *Int. J. Soc. Robot.* **2018**, *11*, 343–358. [CrossRef]
72. Moro, C.; Lin, S.; Nejat, G. Mihailidis: Social robots and seniors: A comparative study on the influence of dynamic social features on human-robot interaction. *Int. J. Soc. Robot.* **2019**, *11*, 5–24. [CrossRef]
73. Portugal, D.; Alvito, P.; Christodoulou, E.; Samaras, G.; Dias, J. A Study on the Deployment of a Service Robot in an Elderly Care Center. *Int. J. Soc. Robot.* **2018**, *11*, 317–341. [CrossRef]
74. Fattal, C.; Leynaert, V.; Laffont, I.; Baillet, A.; Enjalbert, M.; Leroux, C. SAM, an Assistive Robotic Device Dedicated to Helping Persons with Quadriplegia: Usability Study. *Int. J. Soc. Robot.* **2018**, *11*, 89–103. [CrossRef]
75. Zhang, J.; Zhang, H.; Dong, C.; Huang, F.; Liu, Q.; Song, A. Architecture and Design of a Wearable Robotic System for Body Posture Monitoring, Correction, and Rehabilitation Assist. *Int. J. Soc. Robot.* **2019**, *11*, 423–436. [CrossRef]
76. Wang, L.; Du, Z.; Dong, W.; Shen, Y.; Zhao, G. Hierarchical Human Machine Interaction Learning for a Lower Extremity Augmentation Device. *Int. J. Soc. Robot.* **2018**, *11*, 123–139. [CrossRef]
77. PARO Therapeutic Robot. Available online: http://www.parorobots.com/ (accessed on 22 February 2021).
78. Kelly, P.A.; Cox, L.A.; Petersen, S.F.; Gilder, R.E.; Blann, A.E.; Autrey, A.; MacDonell, K. The effect of PARO robotic seals for hospitalized patients with dementia: A feasibility study. *Geriatr. Nurs.* **2021**, *42*, 37–45. [CrossRef]
79. Tavaszi, I.; Nagy, A.S.; Szabo, G.; Fazekas, G. Neglect syndrome in post-stroke conditions. *Int. J. Rehabil. Res.* **2020**. [CrossRef]
80. Jøranson, N.; Olsen, C.; Calogiuri, G.; Ihlebæk, C.; Pedersen, I. Effects on sleep from group activity with a robotic seal for nursing home residents with dementia: A cluster randomized controlled trial. *Int. Psychogeriatrics* **2020**, 1–12. [CrossRef] [PubMed]
81. Kolstad, M.; Yamaguchi, N.; Babic, A.; Nishihara, Y. Integrating Socially Assistive Robots into Japanese Nursing Care. *Stud. Health Technol. Inform.* **2020**, *272*, 183–186. [CrossRef] [PubMed]
82. Jones, C.; Liu, F.; Murfield, J.; Moyle, W. Effects of non-facilitated meaningful activities for people with dementia in long-term care facilities: A systematic review. *Geriatr. Nurs.* **2020**, *41*, 863–871. [CrossRef] [PubMed]
83. Kolstad, M.; Yamaguchi, N.; Babic, A.; Nishihara, Y. Integrating Socially Assistive Robots into Japanese Nursing Care. *Stud. Health Technol. Inform.* **2020**, *270*, 1323–1324. [CrossRef]
84. Geva, N.; Uzefovsky, F.; Levy-Tzedek, S. Touching the social robot PARO reduces pain perception and salivary oxytocin levels. *Sci. Rep.* **2020**, *10*, 1–15. [CrossRef]
85. Pu, L.; Todorovic, M.; Moyle, W.; Jones, C. Using Salivary Cortisol as an Objective Measure of Physiological Stress in People With Dementia and Chronic Pain: A Pilot Feasibility Study. *Biol. Res. Nurs.* **2020**, *22*, 520–526. [CrossRef] [PubMed]

86. Khan, Z.H.; Siddique, A.; Lee, C.W. Robotics Utilization for Healthcare Digitization in Global COVID-19 Management. *Int. J. Environ. Res. Public Health* **2020**, *17*, 3819. [CrossRef] [PubMed]
87. The Strong Robot with the Gentle Touch. Available online: https://www.riken.jp/en/news_pubs/research_news/pr/2015/20150223_2/ (accessed on 22 February 2021).
88. Huijnen, C.A.G.J.; Lexis, M.A.S.; Jansens, R.; De Witte, L.P. Roles, Strengths and Challenges of Using Robots in Interventions for Children with Autism Spectrum Disorder (ASD). *J. Autism Dev. Disord.* **2018**, *49*, 11–21. [CrossRef] [PubMed]
89. Huijnen, C.A.G.J.; Lexis, M.A.S.; Jansens, R.; De Witte, L.P. How to Implement Robots in Interventions for Children with Autism? A Co-creation Study Involving People with Autism, Parents and Professionals. *J. Autism Dev. Disord.* **2017**, *47*, 3079–3096. [CrossRef]
90. Mengoni, S.E.; Irvine, K.; Thakur, D.; Barton, G.; Dautenhahn, K.; Guldberg, K.; Robins, B.; Wellsted, D.; Sharma, S. Feasibility study of a randomised controlled trial to investigate the effectiveness of using a humanoid robot to improve the social skills of children with autism spectrum disorder (Kaspar RCT): A study protocol. *BMJ Open* **2017**, *7*, e017376. [CrossRef] [PubMed]
91. Wood, L.J.; Dautenhahn, K.; Rainer, A.; Robins, B.; Lehmann, H.; Syrdal, D.S. Robot-Mediated Interviews—How Effective Is a Humanoid Robot as a Tool for Interviewing Young Children? *PLoS ONE* **2013**, *8*, e59448. [CrossRef]
92. Giansanti, D. Towards the evolution of the mHealth in mental health with youth: The cyber-space used in psychological rehabilitation is becoming wearable into a pocket. *mHealth* **2020**, *6*, 18. [CrossRef]
93. Giansanti, D.; Monoscalco, L. The cyber-risk in cardiology: Towards an investigation on the self perception among the cardiologists. *mHealth* **2020**. [CrossRef]
94. Giansanti, D.; Monoscalco, L. A smartphone-based survey in mHealth to investigate the introduction of the artificial intelligence into cardiology. *mHealth* **2021**, *7*, 8. [CrossRef]
95. Mejia, C.; Kajikawa, Y. Bibliometric Analysis of Social Robotics Research: Identifying Research Trends and Knowledgebase. *Appl. Sci.* **2017**, *7*, 1316. [CrossRef]
96. Social Robots Market—Growth, Trends, COVID-19 Impact, and Forecasts (2021–2026). Available online: https://www.mordorintelligence.com/industry-reports/social-robots-market (accessed on 22 February 2021).

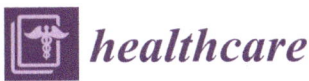

Article

Impacts of Human Robot Proxemics on Human Concentration-Training Games with Humanoid Robots

Li Liu [1], Yangguang Liu [2,*] and Xiao-Zhi Gao [3]

1. College of Digital Technology and Engineering, Ningbo University of Finance and Economics, Ningbo 315175, China; liuli6883@nbufe.edu.cn
2. College of Finance and Information, Ningbo University of Finance and Economics, Ningbo 315175, China
3. School of Computing, University of Eastern Finland, 70210 Kuopio, Finland; xiao-zhi.gao@uef.fi
* Correspondence: liuyangguang@nbufe.edu.cn

Abstract: The use of humanoid robots within a therapeutic role, that is, helping individuals with social disorders, is an emerging field, but it remains unexplored in terms of concentration training. To seamlessly integrate humanoid robots into concentration games, an investigation into the impacts of human robot interactive proxemics on concentration-training games is particularly important. In the case of an epidemic diffusion especially—for example, during the COVID-19 pandemic— HRI games may help in the therapeutic phase, significantly reducing the risk of contagion. In this paper, concentration games were designed by action imitation involving 120 participants to verify the hypothesis. Action-imitation accuracy, the assessment of emotional expression, and a questionnaire were compared with analysis of variance (ANOVA). Experimental results showed that a 2 m distance and left-front orientation for a human and a robot are optimal for human robot interactive concentration training. In addition, females worked better than males did in HRI imitation games. This work supports some valuable suggestions for the development of HRI concentration-training technology, involving the designs of friendlier and more useful robots, and HRI game scenarios.

Keywords: human robot proxemics; human robot interaction; concentration training; psychology response; proxemic distance; nonverbal behavior

Citation: Liu, L.; Liu, Y.; Gao, X.-Z. Impacts of Human Robot Proxemics on Human Concentration-Training Games with Humanoid Robots. *Healthcare* **2021**, *9*, 894. https:// doi.org/10.3390/healthcare9070894

Academic Editor: Daniele Giansanti

Received: 31 May 2021
Accepted: 10 July 2021
Published: 15 July 2021

Publisher's Note: MDPI stays neutral with regard to jurisdictional claims in published maps and institutional affiliations.

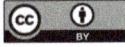

Copyright: © 2021 by the authors. Licensee MDPI, Basel, Switzerland. This article is an open access article distributed under the terms and conditions of the Creative Commons Attribution (CC BY) license (https:// creativecommons.org/licenses/by/ 4.0/).

1. Introduction

Thanks to the advances in robotic technology, human robot interaction (HRI) is popularly used for a variety of applications, including in-store sales [1], entertainment [2], education [3], personal healthcare [4], and therapy [5]. As an increasing amount of the human workforce is replaced by robots, HRI should naturally be widely used in education [2,4]. The application of HRI in education faces many challenges [5], such as how people accept robot partners, how human robot interactive proxemics influence the experiences of humans, and how robots work with humans, such as human co-workers, especially in special-education areas. Human concentration training is an important skill in special education [6]. Imitation learning is an important, widely used method in concentration training, by which an agent tries to mimic an action performed by another [7]. There are four crucial indicators for the assessment of concentration—namely, imitation accuracy, short-term memory, attention stability, and persistence [8–10]. This provides a powerful mechanism whereby knowledge may be transferred between agents (both biological and artificial).

1.1. Imitation Learning

A significant number of studies have been published on imitation learning in animals and humans that state that imitation should be triggered by mirror neurons that are active both during action execution and during perception of one's learning partner performing the same action [7]. They proposed that familiar environments are conducive to stimuli, and imitating should trigger a familiar or unfamiliar response in how a stimulus changes. Stéphane and co-workers found that many sulcus neurons are excited by the actions of specific body parts of an observed human, which seem to be the perfect candidates for the first processing step of imitation [8–10]. Butler indicated neurons in area F5 (a cortical area that contains neurons endowed with mirror properties) that are sensitive to the performance of goal-related actions, e.g., "pushing", "leg lift", and "handshake", and suggested that action imitation can promote the development of social skills [11]. Maurtua and co-workers indicated that humanoid robots can compellingly and autonomously play with humans in educational games, replacing the human teacher during the process [12]. Therefore, action imitation is an excellent candidate for human concentration training. However, imitation is impacted by whether agents belong to the same social group, and by whether the context is competitive cooperation [13,14]. The aim of these previous investigations in HRI was to investigate how humans and robots interact together in a shared physical space while accomplishing a goal [15]. Thus, a human cognizes a robot partner in HRI imitation depending on the physical interaction, distance, actions, and the environment itself.

1.2. HRI Imitation

The crucial consideration for HRI imitation is proxemics, which typically contains the physical (e.g., physical distance and orientation) [16] and psychological (e.g., mutual gaze or willingness) expressions [17] of an interaction. Humans may recognize robots that have no suitable distancing behavior as a threat and obstruction to their social work. Physiological affection is also a crucial factor in HRI games because it directly impacts the willingness of humans to accept robot-executed information, following robot representation [18]. The recognition of emotional expressions and the perception of emotions in general plays a crucial role in social interpersonal communication [19]. Wainer provided a probabilistic framework for psychophysical expression to bridge the gap between these physical and psychological expressions by considering the cognitive experience of each agent in HRI. Robots with appropriately proxemic behaviors might obtain human acceptance well, contributing to their seamless integration into various applications [20]. Jerčić and Lindley suggested that serious games which are carefully designed to take into consideration the elicited physiological arousal might witness better decision-making performance and more positive valence using nonhumanoid-robot partners instead of human ones [21]. Liu showed that embodied nonhumanoid robots are as engaging as humans, eliciting physiological arousal in their human partners [22]. Evidence further indicates that human are sensitive to the environmental cues of cooperative robots, which easily elicits the physiological affection of human partners [23,24]. To the best of our knowledge, there are very few studies on HRI imitation games for human concentration training, and no guidelines exist for the future design of proximity behaviors for robots in concentration training [25,26]. For example, it would be undesirable if human robot proxemics in the HRI games were not suitable, because such behavior comes across as unintelligent and unfriendly [27]. Hence, researchers need to know whether people are likely to assess the distance between the robot and human when they observe them, and which factors can modulate those perceptions [28].

2. Materials
2.1. Human Robot Interactive Game

Current methods to investigate HRI games fall into two categories: behavioral and psychological approaches. For behavioral research, because games are played covering a variety of activities, no precise definition of gameplay has been presented [29]. Many methods deal with gameplay and research this field differently in terms of their special purposes. Games may exhibit two different representations: active and passive learning. All forms of gameplay need human interest, concentration, and mental activity [30]. Psychological research on HRI games involves many factors, such as preferences, comfort, security, and happiness. Some research related to HRI games was performed, but the studies mainly focused on the relationships between people and their robot players [31]. There have been some studies on the effects in collaborative HRI games, and the design of a context-aware proxemic planner which aims to improve a robot's social behavior by adapting its distance management [32].

2.2. Human Robot Proxemics

Impact factors of HRI concentration-training games usually contain human robot interactive distance, proxemic direction, robot size and appearance, and the environment [27–29,33–35]. The first two factors significantly influence people's experiences with and perceptions of a human-like robot in HRI games [6]. Physical interpersonal distances should conform to societal norms (relative distances between people) that are expressed in four distinct zones, i.e., intimate space, personal space, social space, and public space, as shown in Figure 1 [36]. The space between intimate and personal distance is called personal space (ranging from 0.46 to 1.22 m). The space between social and personal distance is called the social space (ranging from 1.2 to 3.7 m). The space within public distance is called the public space (ranging from 3.7 m to infinite).

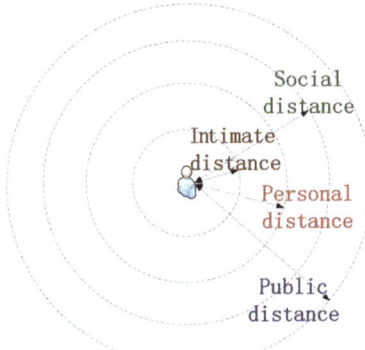

Figure 1. Relationships between interpersonal position and sensory experiences.

Human proxemic behavior contains physical and psychological distance. There are some papers related to interpersonal distances [37] and the fixed distances among human groups [38].

2.3. Human Concentration Training

Concentration is essential for humans. It is giving attention to a task, which is good for performing at one's best while not being affected by irrelevant external and internal stimuli [39–42]. External stimuli involve the external environment, context, and voices. Concentration or attention is very important in sport psychology [43]. It is evidently difficult to study the processes of some people because of the lack of concentration [44]. The use of robots in the concentration-training context offers students new effective learning strategies in HRI spaces through a personalized and unique experience. With suitable interaction schemes, the usage of HRI concentration-training games could improve participant performance [45].

2.4. Hypotheses

Some promising studies in human robot interaction have explored proxemic behavior, as described in the last section. These studies show promising evidence that people express proxemic preferences when they are interacting with robots [2,29,30,44], but comprehensive theoretical models or experimental results of physical and psychological distancing are needed to guide the design of proxemic behaviors for robots. We formed three hypotheses for human robot proxemics in concentration-training games based on the models that presented findings from human robot interaction studies [27,36,37,46].

Hypothesis 1. *Following perceptual models of human robot proxemics [44], outcomes are derived from nonverbal behaviors, which explains the impacts of human proxemics on the effectiveness of HRI, assuming that the physical distance between human and robot is face-to-face during HRI imitation play.*

Hypothesis 2. *Following human proxemics [46], to understand how people physically and psychologically relate to robots compared to other humans, direction has little effect on HRI concentration-training games. Therefore, direction has little impact on the accuracy rate of action imitation, and the right-front direction has a slightly larger effect for face-to-face HRI games.*

Hypothesis 3. *Following existing studies of human proxemics, the best HRI distance for face-to-face, front-on imitation games is thought to be 1–2 m, and the effectiveness of HRI imitation games, e.g., comfortability and fun, is significantly impacted.*

In the next section, a controlled laboratory experiment is described in which these hypotheses were evaluated in a human robot interaction scenario.

3. Methods

A controlled laboratory experiment was designed to explore how human robot proxemics influence HRI concentration training by action-imitation games in which a tester demonstrates random movements, and participants are to immediately repeating them (approximately). Experimental datasets, the procedure, measurements, results, and participant information are described below.

3.1. Experimental Conditions

The experiments consisted of a game scenario involving a participant, a tester, and an operator. The tester could be either a human or a semiautonomous robot that was manipulated by the operator. The controlled-play scenario was in an enclosed laboratory with controlled light that was free from outside distractions. The width of the experimental site was 11 m, and the length was 13 m. During the game, the participant sat on a chair against the wall facing the tester, who could not stand up or turn. The tester was fixed face to face with the participant, and the directions in front of the participant were set from left to right as $-45°, 0°$, and $45°$. The distance between participant and tester was divided into seven different steps (from 0.5 to 3.5 m with a step of 0.5 m) and three different spatial directions. There were 21 position tags set on the floor by distance and direction between participant and tester that were numbered from 1 to 21, as shown in Figure 2.

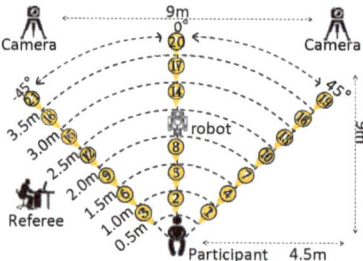

Figure 2. Experimental setup of concentration-training games with a humanoid robot.

The experimental equipment was one laptop, one humanoid robot, two cameras, one chair, and one game positioning tag. The humanoid robot was controlled to move semiautonomously by an operator, executing nonverbal action like a human. The testers were a human tester and a humanoid-robot tester.

3.2. Participation

The participants were 120 students with an age range from 17 to 20 invited by a local university: 60 females and 60 males. All students could perform normal imitation behaviors according to the testers; they had no difficulty in movement and were accepting of the game.

3.3. Experimental Design

In our experiments, every participant would play random action-imitation games with a tester to evaluate concentration. The imitation games comprised two modules for every participant, namely, playing with the human tester and with the humanoid-robot tester. Researchers conducted two modules of imitation games for every participant at every experimental position (from 1 to 21), which alternately started with the human or robot player. Each participant needed to successively perform three random continuous actions mimicking the tester, including left or right-leg lifting, left or right-hand raising, and raising both hands. After the tester finished executing an action, the participant had to mimic the action for no more than 3 s.

A points system was utilized to judge whether the participant would win the game, and the rules of the game were as follows. One point was awarded if the participant accurately mimicked the action within the specified time; otherwise, no point was awarded. The maximal score for one participant was 84 points. If the participant got 76 points or more, they won the game. At the end of the game, each participant was asked to complete a questionnaire containing eight open-ended questions. Each question was graded on a scale of 1 to 5, representing "strongly dislike" to "strongly like." After answering the questionnaire, the game ended, and the next participant played the game [47].

3.4. Experimental Procedure

Only a tester, a participant, and a referee were present for the game. When the experiment started, the participant was asked to sit down and direct their concentration to the operator, who introduced the rules of the human–human interactive (HHI) concentration game [31,36]. When the operator finished the introduction of the game, they confirmed that the participant had clearly understood the rules of the game. Then, the participant began to play the imitation game.

Every participant played with a human tester and a robot tester. In order to achieve the objective and reasonable experimental results, every participant played with the same tester for 2 rounds with a sequence of $(1, 2, 3, \cdots, 21)$ and an opposite sequence of $(21, 20, 19, \cdots, 1)$. Random actions were determined by the tester regardless of sequence. Random imitation games mainly related to the choice of body posture and not the sequence.

3.5. Measurement

There were three independent manipulated variables in our experiments: (1) humanoid-robot size, (2) humanoid-robot appearance, and (3) random actions of the tester. All independent variables were operated by the tester. The dependent variables involved in the participant measurements related to imitation accuracy, comfortability, and fun were proxemic distance and direction. The imitation games with the human tester were compared to those with the robot tester by using the combination methods of imitation accuracy, assessment of emotional expression, and questionnaires. The impacts of distance and direction on the imitation games were explored, thereby finding the optimal human robot proxemics for HRI imitation games.

4. Results

Analysis of the experimental results was related to the physical distance between and orientations of participants and the tester using analysis of variance (ANOVA) [37,39]. All experimental results were processed and analyzed by SPSS software. Analysis of imitation accuracy was mixed-effects repeated measures ANOVA, where physical distance and direction were random effects, but imitation actions and robot appearance conditions were fixed effects. The two other independent variables, participant gender and age, were fixed effects. Psychological distance was analyzed using the questionnaire method.

4.1. Proxemic Distance and Direction

Physical distance: experimental results demonstrated the main effect of physical distance on the imitation-accuracy rate of HHI or HRI games. The proximity distance between participant and tester significantly influenced HHI imitation games, $F(1,6) = 3.35, p < 0.01$, as shown in Figure 3a.

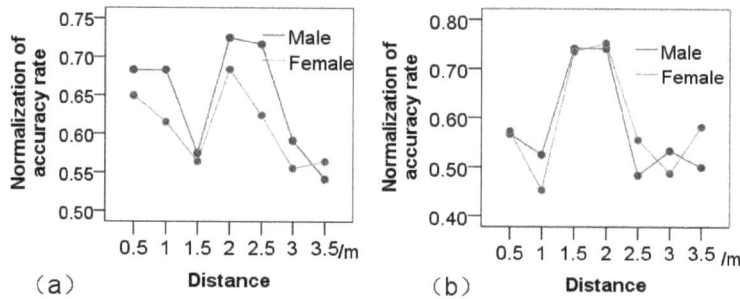

Figure 3. Comparison of the normalization of accuracy rate at different distances for action imitation. (**a**) HHI games; (**b**) HRI games.

At seven different orientations at 2 m, the highest imitation-accuracy rate was achieved, $F(13,804) = 2.98, p < 0.01$. Beyond 3 m, the accuracy rate was linearly decreased. At the same time, the proximity's influence on imitation-accuracy rate was analyzed. Analysis proved that proximity significantly influenced the accuracy rate of the HRI imitation game: $F(1,6) = 12.52, p < 0.001$, as shown in Figure 3b.

As in the HHI game, the highest accuracy rate of the imitation game was at the physical distance of 2 m, $F(13,804) = 3.484, p < 0.001$. The distance between the participant and the human or robot tester therefore had an obviously significant influence on the concentration-training game. Therefore, the experimental results confirmed the hypothesis that, at 2 m, participants have the best imitation accuracy. This was the case for both HHI and HRI imitation games, as shown in Figure 3.

Furthermore, the influence of gender on the concentration-training game was also analyzed. In the HHI game, experimental results demonstrated that male participants had slightly higher accuracy than female participants. The influence of gender on the accuracy of the concentration games was small: $F(1,804) = 1.239, p > 0.05$, as shown in Figure 4a. In HRI games, results demonstrated no significant difference between males and females: $F(1,804) = 0.077, p > 0.05$, as shown in Figure 4b. At 2 m distance, male and female participants were almost equally accurate.

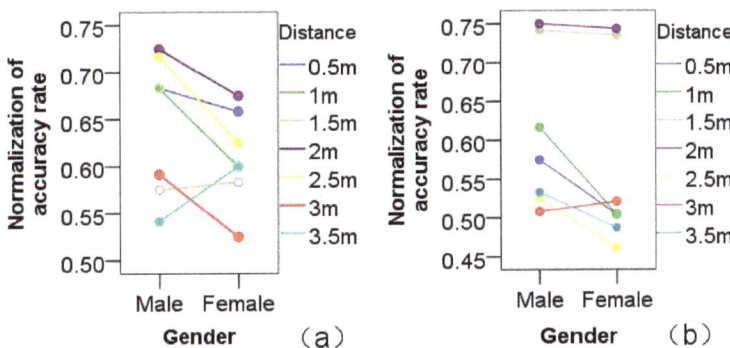

Figure 4. Distance analysis: effect of distance on action-imitation games played by participants of different genders in different game scenarios. (**a**) HHI games; (**b**) HRI games.

Proxemics direction: results showed that direction is another significant factor that influences concentration games. In HHI games, direction was the main impact factor. Results showed that there were different accuracy levels when the tester was in different directions: $F(2, 2457) = 2.899, p < 0.05$. The accuracy of the HHI games was higher when the tester was at $-45°$, rather than at other directions: $F(2, 360) = 2.589, p < 0.05$, as shown in Figure 5a. In HRI games, results showed that direction was an impact factor, but not significantly: $F(2, 2425) = 1.699, p > 0.05$, as shown in Figure 5b. According to analysis, the HRI game's results were similar for $-45°$ and $45°$. At the same time, males had an obviously better accuracy rate than that of females for any direction, especially in HRI games. Analysis confirmed Hypothesis 1, and the direction of $-45°$ was more conducive to the face-to-face HRI game.

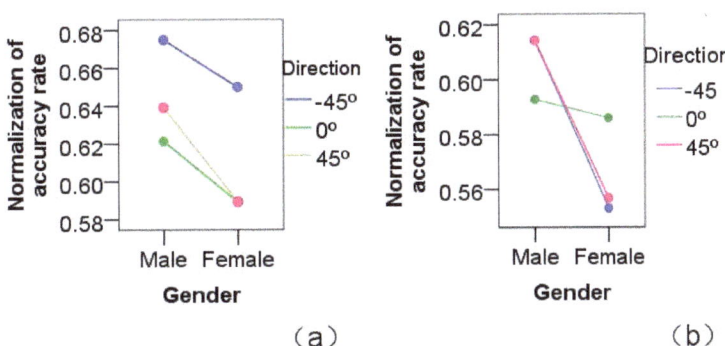

Figure 5. Direction analysis: the effects on action-imitation games of gender, different directions, and different game scenarios. (**a**) HHI games; (**b**) HRI games.

Additionally, comparative results of the influences of direction on HHI and HRI imitation games are shown in Figure 6a,b, respectively. By comparatively analyzing the experimental results of the two different modules of imitation games, the impact of direction on HRI games was shown to be less than on HHI games. Experimental results showed that Hypothesis 2 was valid.

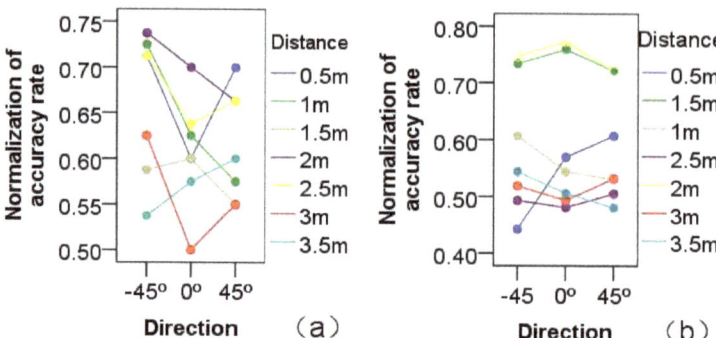

Figure 6. The effects of different proxemic distances and different directions. (**a**) HHI games; (**b**) HRI games.

4.2. Perception of Students' Emotional Expression

Researchers discussed students' imitation accuracy in the interaction games with humans, and compared the results with those obtained by students playing with the humanoid robot. During the whole experimental procedure, the participants were videotaped. There were various types of nonverbal social behaviors and emotional responses to winning or losing in a game. In this section, we analyze the emotional responses from selected recordings of the participants that were taken under HHI or HRI conditions by third-party judges. A judge's task was to evaluate via the video clips whether a participant had won or lost the game. By this method, the expressiveness of the participant would objectively be estimated in different experimental conditions, and indicate whether participants were more expressive via a more correct estimation.

Forty student observers were invited to judge whether participants won or lost games by observing their emotions in the video clips. The student observers were divided into four groups. Each group was invited into a classroom where the representative frames from video clips were projected onto a wall. Six different frames were shown in order at a time. In 5 s, observers had to make a judgment and write the score on a piece of paper.

The researchers analyzed the data from the two different scenarios to study significant effects for the concentration games by comparing judgment accuracy. For collected data in various experiments, the two main scenarios of interest (human and robot testers) were statistically compared with independent-sample t-tests. The judgmental-accuracy rate of the observers for the HHI game (M = 0.87) was slightly higher than that for the HRI game (M = 0.80), t (553) = 5.01, $p < 0.001$. Therefore, participants were more expressive in HHI concentration games than in HRI games. The expressions of female and male students were compared. Male students (M = 0.90) were more expressive than female students (M = 0.81) in HHI games, as shown in Figure 7. However, in HRI games, the judgment accuracy of the male participants was similar to that of female participants. Results showed that male students playing with humans were more expressive than female students in the HHI imitation games. However, in HRI imitation games, the male students playing with humanoid robots were as expressive as female students.

In addition, the effect of proxemic distance on a participant's expressions during the game was studied. The accuracy of judgments for participants' 297 emotional expressions at different distances in HHI and HRI games are summarized in Tables 1 and 2, respectively. Accuracy of judgment at the 2 m distance was higher (($M = 0.35$), F (1, 6) =12.87, $p > 0.001$) than that at other distances in the HHI games. Similarly to HHI games, the percentage of judgmental accuracy rate was higher (($M = 0.39$), $F(1, 6) = 14.52, p > 0.001$) at the 2 m distance than that in other distances in the HRI games. The percentage of judgmental-accuracy rate demonstrates that the participants' expressions at the 2 m distance in the HRI game were more obvious than that at the 2 m distance in the HHI game. Thus, the effect of proxemic distance on the emotion expression in the HRI games was more obvious than that in the HHI games. The effect of proxemic direction on participant expressions during the game was also studied. The accuracy of judgment showed that different directions had little effect on the expression effect. In the next section, the psychological response is analyzed by questionnaire.

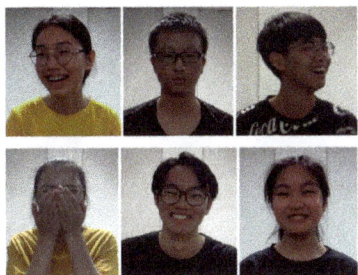

Figure 7. Representative stills of undergraduates' reactions after winning or losing a game while playing with a human (**top**) or robot (**bottom**).

In the questionnaire investigation, our analysis showed that students preferred playing with humans (M = 0.56) over playing with robots $(M = 0.48), t(90) = 8.01, p < 0.001$, as shown in Figure 8. Female participants disclosed a marginal preference for a human tester over a robot tester, $F(1, 129) = 5.21, p < 0.05$. Our analysis further confirmed that proxemic distance had a more significant effect on participants' play psychology in HRI games, $F(1, 6) = 11.15, p < 0.001$ than that in the HHI games, $F(1, 6) = 15.23, p < 0.001$. The range of 1.5 to 2 m distance was most people's choice, as shown in Figure 9.

Table 1. Numbers of occurrences of emotional expressions in HHI games.

Responsive Category	Emotional Expression	0.5 m	1 m	1.5 m	2 m	2.5 m	3 m	3.5 m
Win	Smile	200	147	88	94	126	111	134
	Laugh	41	79	116	139	108	86	77
	Winning gesture	2	5	5	9	8	5	0
	Total positive features	243	231	209	242	242	202	211
Loss	Frown	114	86	87	51	63	87	96
	Closing eyes	5	44	62	55	52	66	55
	Head down	0	0	2	1	2	4	2
	Total negative features	119	130	151	107	117	157	153

Table 2. Numbers of occurrences of emotional expressions in HRI games.

Responsive Category	Emotional Expression	0.5 m	1 m	1.5 m	2 m	2.5 m	3 m	3.5 m
Win	Smile	135	124	150	171	89	99	123
	Laugh	54	72	105	94	83	85	59
	Winning gesture	6	6	8	4	5	0	3
	Total positive features	195	202	263	269	177	184	185
Loss	Frown brown	117	105	36	24	116	114	126
	Closing eyes	39	49	57	63	62	57	45
	Head down	6	2	2	2	4	3	3
	Total negative features	162	156	95	89	182	174	174

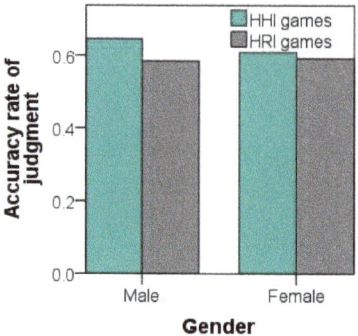

Figure 8. Accuracy rates of judgments for participants winning or losing by evaluating their emotional expressions in HHI and HRI games.

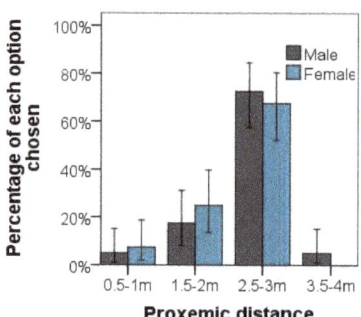

Figure 9. Presentation of selection results for each distance chosen by all student participants.

According to analysis, 2 m was the optimal proxemic distance in both HHI and HRI games. Analysis verified the hypothesis that 2 m distance was the best human robot distance for both HHI and HRI concentration-training games. Direction had little influence on the psychological experience in HRI games $F(1,2) = 2.05, p = ns$, as in HHI games $F(1,2) = 1.12, p = ns$. In summary, experimental results show that Hypothesis 3 is valid.

Various methods of analysis showed that the experimental results were continuous. The combined evidence of imitation accuracy, emotional-expression assessments and questionnaire investigation agreed with the hypothesis.

5. Conclusions

This paper provided a new approach to assess human concentration training by using an imitation game with a humanoid robot. The effects of proxemic distance and direction on the concentration-training game were analyzed with HHI and HRI imitation games. In total, 120 participants who were 18-year-old students from the same university were invited to play the imitation games.

On the basis of the findings, this study contributes to HRI research in the following ways.

- Direction for imitation is less important for robot trainers than for human trainers, so in a classroom, a robot may be placed at any angle in front of the learner.
- Suitable distance is good for trusting a robot, which is vital for subjects' willingness to play with the robot.
- The different physiological effects in humans collaborating with a robot partner and a human partner were comparatively analyzed.

- Students of different genders responded to HRI and HHI games differently, which indicated that female students had more interest in playing the imitation game with a humanoid robot than male students did.
- Students felt that playing with people was similar to playing with humanoid robots.

To promote HRI instead of HHI games in human concentration training, future research should explicitly consider individual differences, such as cultural background and age, during the HRI game-design process. Humans are more interested in using HRI games because of an attractive robot implemented with smart objects. Overall, this study could inform the practice of HRI games, and the design of friendly and useful robots.

Author Contributions: L.L. conceived the study and care about conceptualization, data curation, analysis, methodology, interpretation of data and writing draft. Y.L., X.-Z.G. took care about data curation, analysis, methodology, interpretation of data and writing review and editing. All authors have read and agreed to the published version of the manuscript.

Funding: This work was supported by the Zhejiang Philosophy and Social Science Planning Project (Grant No.19NDJC103YB), the Humanities and Social Science Research Youth Foundation of the Ministry of Education (Grant No.19YJC880053), the Natural Science Foundation of Zhejiang province (Grant No. LQ18F010008).

Institutional Review Board Statement: The study was conducted according to the guidelines of the Declaration of Helsinki, and approved by the Research Ethics Board of the Ningbo University of Finace and Economics (20180028, approved 1 December 2018).

Informed Consent Statement: Informed consent was obtained from all subjects involved in the study.

Data Availability Statement: The data presented in this study are available on request from the corresponding author. The data are not publicly available due to privacy reasons.

Acknowledgments: All the participants are gratefully acknowledged.

Conflicts of Interest: The authors declare no conflict of interest. The funders had no role in the design of the study; in the collection, analyses, or interpretation of data; in the writing of the manuscript, or in the decision to publish the results.

References

1. Gross, H.M.; Boehme, H.; Schroeter, C.; Mueller, S.; Koenig, A.; Einhorn, E.; Martin, C.; Merten, M.; Bley, A. TOOMAS: Interactive Shopping Guide Robots in Everyday Use—Final Implementation and Experiences from Long-Term Field Trials. In Proceedings of the 2009 IEEE/RSJ International Conference on Intelligent Robots and Systems, St. Louis, MO, USA, 10–15 October 2009; pp. 2005–2012.
2. Broadbent, E.; Kuo, I.H.; Lee, Y.; Rabindran, J.; Kerse, N.; Stafford, R.; Macdonald, B. Attitudes and Reactions to a Healthcare Robot. *Telemed. J. E-Health Off. J. Am. Telemed. Assoc.* **2010**, *16*, 608–613. [CrossRef] [PubMed]
3. Hyun, E.; Yoon, H.; Son, S. Relationships between User Experiences and Children's Perceptions of the Education Robot. In Proceedings of the 5th ACM/IEEE International Conference on Human-Robot Interaction, Osaka, Japan, 2–5 March 2010; pp. 199–200.
4. De Jong, M.; Zhang, K.; Roth, A.M.; Rhodes, T.; Schmucker, R.; Zhou, C.; Ferreira, S.; Cartucho, J.; Veloso, M.M. Towards a Robust Interactive and Learning Social Robot. In Proceedings of the 17th International Conference on Autonomous Agents and MultiAgent Systems, AAMAS 2018, Stockholm, Sweden, 10–15 July 2018; André, E., Koenig, S., Dastani, M., Sukthankar, G., Eds.; pp. 883–891.
5. Ayerbe, M.; Gonzalez, D.; Jimenez, F.; Guerrero, E.; Correal, A. AIO robot: A EDI modular robotic dramatization platform. In Proceedings of the 2017 18th International Conference on Advanced Robotics (ICAR), Hong Kong, China, 10–12 July 2017; pp. 262–268. [CrossRef]
6. Kaptein, F.; Broekens, J.; Hindriks, K.V.; Neerincx, M.A. Personalised self-explanation by robots: The role of goals versus beliefs in robot-action explanation for children and adults. In Proceedings of the 26th IEEE International Symposium on Robot and Human Interactive Communication, RO-MAN 2017, Lisbon, Portugal, 28 August–1 September 2017; pp. 676–682. [CrossRef]
7. Pacchierotti, E.; Christensen, H.; Jensfelt, P. Human-robot embodied interaction in hallway settings: A pilot user study. In Proceedings of the IEEE International Workshop on Robot and Human Interactive Communication, Nashville, TN, USA, 13–15 August 2005; Volume 2005, pp. 164–171. [CrossRef]
8. Stéphane, R.; Salesse, R.; Ludovic, M.; Del-Monte, J.; Schmidt, R.; Varlet, M.; Bardy, B.; Boulenger, J.P.; Capdevielle, D. Social priming enhances interpersonal synchronization and feeling of connectedness towards schizophrenia patients. *Sci. Rep.* **2015**, *5*, 8156. [CrossRef]

9. Jensen, W.; Hansen, S.; Knoche, H. Knowing You, Seeing Me: Investigating User Preferences in Drone-Human Acknowledgement. In Proceedings of the 2018 CHI Conference on Human Factors in Computing Systems, Montreal, QC, Canada, 21–26 April 2018; pp. 1–12. [CrossRef]
10. Rizzolatti, G.; Craighero, L. The Mirror-Neuron System. *Annu. Rev. Neurosci.* **2004**, *27*, 169–192. [CrossRef] [PubMed]
11. Butler, J.; Agah, A. Psychological Effects of Behavior Patterns of a Mobile Personal Robot. *Auton. Robot.* **2001**, *10*, 185–202. [CrossRef]
12. Maurtua, I.; Fernandez, I.; Kildal, J.; Susperregi, L.; Tellaeche, A.; Ibarguren, A. Enhancing safe human-robot collaboration through natural multimodal communication. In Proceedings of the 2016 IEEE 21st International Conference on Emerging Technologies and Factory Automation (ETFA), Berlin, Germany, 6–9 September 2016; pp. 1–8. [CrossRef]
13. Song, B.; Gao, M. A Decentralized Context-aware Cross-domain Authorization Scheme for Pervasive Computing. In Proceedings of the 8th International Conference on Networks, Communication and Computing, ICNCC 2019, Luoyang, China, 13–15 December 2019; pp. 28–31. [CrossRef]
14. Bethel, C.; Salomon, K.; Murphy, R.; Burke, J. Survey of Psychophysiology Measurements Applied to Human-Robot Interaction. In Proceedings of the RO-MAN 2007—The 16th IEEE International Symposium on Robot and Human Interactive Communication, Jeju, Korea, 26–29 August 2007; pp. 732–737. [CrossRef]
15. Kim, Y.; Mutlu, B. How social distance shapes human–robot interaction. *Int. J. Hum. Comput. Stud.* **2014**, *72*, 783–795. [CrossRef]
16. van den Brule, R.; Dotsch, R.; Bijlstra, G.; Wigboldus, D.; Haselager, P. Do Robot Performance and Behavioral Style affect Human Trust?: A Multi-Method Approach. *Int. J. Soc. Robot.* **2014**, *6*, 519–531. [CrossRef]
17. De Santis, A.; Siciliano, B.; Luca, A.; Bicchi, A. An atlas of physical human-robot interaction. *Mech. Mach. Theory* **2008**, *43*, 253–270. [CrossRef]
18. Desai, M.; Kaniarasu, P.; Medvedev, M.; Steinfeld, A. Impact of robot failures and feedback on real-time trust. In Proceedings of the 2013 8th ACM/IEEE International Conference on Human-Robot Interaction (HRI), Tokyo, Japan, 3–6 March 2013. [CrossRef]
19. Burgoon, J.; Bonito, J.; Bengtsson, B.; Cederberg, C.; Lundeberg, M.; Allspach, L. Interactivity in human-computer interaction: A study of credibility, understanding, and influence. *Comput. Hum. Behav.* **2000**, *16*, 553–574. [CrossRef]
20. Wainer, J.; Dautenhahn, K.; Robins, B.; Amirabdollahian, F. A Pilot Study with a Novel Setup for Collaborative Play of the Humanoid Robot KASPAR with Children with Autism. *Int. J. Soc. Robot.* **2014**, *6*, 45–65. [CrossRef]
21. Jerčić, P.; Wen, W.; Hagelbäck, J.; Sundstedt, V. The Effect of Emotions and Social Behavior on Performance in a Collaborative Serious Game Between Humans and Autonomous Robots. *Int. J. Soc. Robot.* **2017**, *10*, 115–129. [CrossRef]
22. Liu, P.; Liu, T.; Shi, J.; Wang, X.; Yin, Z.; Zhao, C. Aspect level sentiment classification with unbiased attention and target enhanced representations. In Proceedings of the 35th Annual ACM Symposium on Applied Computing, Brno, Czech Republic, 30 March–3 April 2020; pp. 843–850. [CrossRef]
23. Robinette, P.; Li, W.; Allen, R.; Howard, A.; Wagner, A. Overtrust of Robots in Emergency Evacuation Scenarios. In Proceedings of the 2016 11th ACM/IEEE International Conference on Human-Robot Interaction (HRI), Christchurch, New Zealand, 7–10 March 2016. [CrossRef]
24. Lin, Y.; Min, H.; Zhou, H.; Pei, F. A Human-Robot-Environment Interactive Reasoning Mechanism for Object Sorting Robot. *IEEE Trans. Cogn. Dev. Syst.* **2017**. [CrossRef]
25. Robins, B.; Dautenhahn, K. Tactile Interactions with a Humanoid Robot: Novel Play Scenario Implementations with Children with Autism. *Int. J. Soc. Robot.* **2014**, *6*, 397–415. [CrossRef]
26. Chin, K.Y.; Hong, Z.W.; Chen, Y.L. Impact of Using an Educational Robot-Based Learning System on Students' Motivation in Elementary Education. *IEEE Trans. Learn. Technol.* **2014**, *7*, 333–345. [CrossRef]
27. Yilmazyildiz, S.; Read, R.; Belpeame, T.; Verhelst, W. Review of Semantic-Free Utterances in Social Human–Robot Interaction. *Int. J. Hum. Comput. Interact.* **2016**, *32*, 63–85. [CrossRef]
28. Zaga, C.; Lohse, M.; Truong, K.P.; Evers, V. The Effect of a Robot's Social Character on Children's Task Engagement: Peer Versus Tutor. In *Social Robotics*; Tapus, A., André, E., Martin, J.C., Ferland, F., Ammi, M., Eds.; Springer International Publishing: Cham, Switzerland , 2015; pp. 704–713.
29. Williams, T.; Briggs, P.; Scheutz, M. Covert Robot-Robot Communication: Human Perceptions and Implications for Human-Robot Interaction. *J. Hum. Robot Interact.* **2015**, *4*, 24–49. [CrossRef]
30. Ross Mead, A.A.; Matarić, M.J. *Representations of Proxemic Behavior for Human-Machine Interaction*; Workshop, NordiCHI: Copenhagen, Denmark, 2012.
31. Feil-Seifer, D.; Mataric, M. Automated Detection and Classification of Positive vs. Negative Robot Interactions with Children with Autism Using Distance-Based Features. In Proceedings of the 6th International Conference on Human-Robot Interaction, Lausanne, Switzerland, 8–11 March 2011; Association for Computing Machinery: New York, NY, USA, 2011; pp. 323–330. [CrossRef]
32. Van Oosterhout, T.; Visser, A.O.T. A Visual Method for Robot Proxemics Measurements. In *Proceedings of Metrics for Human-Robot Interaction, a Workshop at ACM/IEEE HRI 2008*; University of Hertfordshire: Hatfield, UK, 2008; pp. 61–68.
33. Bravo Sanchez, F.; Correal, A.; Guerrero, E. Interactive Drama With Robots for Teaching Non-Technical Subjects. *J. Hum. Robot. Interact.* **2017**, *6*, 48. [CrossRef]
34. Brown, L.; Howard, A. Engaging children in math education using a socially interactive humanoid robot. *IEEE-RAS Int. Conf. Humanoid Robot.* **2015**, *2015*, 183–188. [CrossRef]

35. Bouker, J.; Scarlatos, A. Investigating the impact on fluid intelligence by playing N-Back games with a kinesthetic modality. In Proceedings of the 2013 10th International Conference and Expo on Emerging Technologies for a Smarter World (CEWIT), Melville, NY, USA, 21–22 October 2013; pp. 1–3. [CrossRef]
36. Silva, M.P.; do Nascimento Silva, V.; Chaimowicz, L. Dynamic Difficulty Adjustment through an Adaptive AI. In Proceedings of the 14th Brazilian Symposium on Computer Games and Digital Entertainment, SBGames 2015, Piauí, Brazil, 11–13 November 2015; Rodrigues, M.A.F., de Carvalho, F.G., de Vasconcellos, M.S., Eds.; IEEE Computer Society: Piscataway, NJ, USA, 2015; pp. 173–182. [CrossRef]
37. Araujo, V.; Mendez, D.; Gonzalez, A. A Novel Approach to Working Memory Training Based on Robotics and AI. *Information* **2019**, *10*, 350. [CrossRef]
38. Mead, R.; Atrash, A.; Mataric, M.J. Automated Proxemic Feature Extraction and Behavior Recognition: Applications in Human-Robot Interaction. *I. J. Soc. Robot.* **2013**, *5*, 367–378. [CrossRef]
39. Wood, L.J.; Robins, B.; Lakatos, G.; Syrdal, D.S.; Zaraki, A.; Dautenhahn, K. Developing a protocol and experimental setup for using a humanoid robot to assist children with autism to develop visual perspective taking skills. *Paladyn* **2019**, *10*, 167–179. [CrossRef]
40. Frank, M.R.; Autor, D.; Bessen, J.E.; Brynjolfsson, E.; Cebrian, M.; Deming, D.J.; Feldman, M.; Groh, M.; Lobo, J.; Moro, E.; et al. Toward understanding the impact of artificial intelligence on labor. *Proc. Natl. Acad. Sci. USA* **2019**, *116*, 6531–6539. [CrossRef] [PubMed]
41. Vázquez, M.; Carter, E.J.; McDorman, B.; Forlizzi, J.; Steinfeld, A.; Hudson, S.E. Towards Robot Autonomy in Group Conversations: Understanding the Effects of Body Orientation and Gaze. In Proceedings of the 2017 ACM/IEEE International Conference on Human-Robot Interaction, HRI 2017, Vienna, Austria, 6–9 March 2017; Mutlu, B., Tscheligi, M., Weiss, A., Young, J.E., Eds.; ACM: New York, NY, USA, 2017; pp. 42–52. [CrossRef]
42. De Graaf, M.M.A.; Malle, B.F. People's Explanations of Robot Behavior Subtly Reveal Mental State Inferences. In Proceedings of the 14th ACM/IEEE International Conference on Human-Robot Interaction, HRI 2019, Daegu, Korea, 11–14 March 2019; pp. 239–248. [CrossRef]
43. Torabi, F.; Warnell, G.; Stone, P. Adversarial Imitation Learning from State-Only Demonstrations. In Proceedings of the 18th International Conference on Autonomous Agents and MultiAgent Systems, Montreal, QC, Canada, 13–17 May 2019; International Foundation for Autonomous Agents and Multiagent Systems: Richland, SC, USA, 2019; pp. 2229–2231.
44. Berinsky, A.J.; Huber, G.A.; Lenz, G.S. Evaluating Online Labor Markets for Experimental Research: Amazon.com's Mechanical Turk. *Political Anal.* **2012**, *20*, 351–368. [CrossRef]
45. Pan, Y.; Steed, A. A Comparison of Avatar-, Video-, and Robot-Mediated Interaction on Users' Trust in Expertise. *Front. Robot. AI* **2016**, *3*, 12. [CrossRef]
46. Takayama, L.; Pantofaru, C. Influences on Proxemic Behaviors in Human-Robot Interaction. In Proceedings of the 2009 IEEE/RSJ International Conference on Intelligent Robots and Systems, St. Louis, MO, USA, 10–15 October 2009; pp. 5495–5502.
47. Mead, R.; Mataric, M.J. A Probabilistic Framework for Autonomous Proxemic Control in Situated and Mobile Human-Robot Interaction. In *Proceedings of the Seventh Annual ACM/IEEE International Conference on Human-Robot Interaction*; Association for Computing Machinery: New York, NY, USA, 2012; pp. 193–194. [CrossRef]

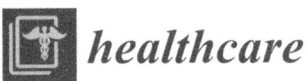

Article

The Social Robot and the Digital Physiotherapist: Are We Ready for the Team Play?

Rossella Simeoni [1], Federico Colonnelli [1], Veronica Eutizi [1], Matteo Marchetti [1], Elena Paolini [1], Valentina Papalini [1], Alessio Punturo [1], Alice Salvò [1], Nicoletta Scipinotti [1], Christian Serpente [1], Emanuele Barbini [1], Riccardo Troscia [1], Giovanni Maccioni [2] and Daniele Giansanti [2,*]

[1] Faculty of Medicine and Surgery, Università Cattolica del Sacro Cuore, San Martino al Cimino, 01100 Viterbo, Italy; rossella.simeoni.1955@gmail.com (R.S.); federico.colonnelli@hotmail.com (F.C.); veronica.eutizi.univ.catt.21@gmail.com (V.E.); matteo.marchetti.univ.catt.21@gmail.com (M.M.); elena.paolini.univ.catt.21@gmail.com (E.P.); valentina.papalini.univ.catt.21@hotmail.com (V.P.); alessio.punturo.univ.catt.21@hotmail.com (A.P.); alice.salvo.univ.catt.21@hotmail.com (A.S.); n.scipinotti.univ.catt@hotmail.com (N.S.); c.serpente.univ.catt@hotmail.com (C.S.); emanuele.barbini.univ.catt.21@hotmail.com (E.B.); r.troscia.univ.catt@hotmail.com (R.T.)
[2] Centre Tisp, Istituto Superiore di Sanità, 00161 Rome, Italy; giovanni.maccioni@iss.it
* Correspondence: daniele.giansanti@iss.it; Tel.: +39-06-4990-2701

Abstract: *Motivation*: We are witnessing two phenomena. The first is that the physiotherapist is increasingly becoming a figure that must interact with Digital Health. On the other hand, social robots through research are improving more and more in the aspects of social interaction thanks also to artificial intelligence and becoming useful in rehabilitation processes. It begins to become strategic to investigate the intersections between these two phenomena. *Objective*: Therefore, we set ourselves the goal of investigating the consensus and opinion of physiotherapists around the introduction of social robots in clinical practice both in rehabilitation and assistance. *Procedure*: An electronic survey has been developed focused on social robot-based rehabilitation and assistance and has been submitted to subjects focused on physiotherapy sciences to investigate their opinion and their level of consent regarding the use of the social robot in rehabilitation and assistance. Two samples of subjects were recruited: the first group (156 participating subjects, 79 males, 77 females, mean age 24.3 years) was in the training phase, and the second (167 participating subjects, 86 males, 81 females, mean age 42.4 years) group was involved in the work processes. An electronic feedback form was also submitted to investigate the acceptance of the proposed methodology. *Results*: The survey showed a consistency of the results between the two samples from which interesting considerations emerge. Contrary to stereotypes that report how AI-based devices put jobs at risk, physiotherapists are not afraid of these devices. The subjects involved in the study believe the following: (a) social robots can be reliable co-workers but will remain a complementary device; (b) their role will be of the utmost importance as an operational manager in their use and in performance monitoring; (c) these devices will allow an increase in working capacity and facilitate integration. All those involved in the study believe that the proposed electronic survey has proved to be a useful and effective tool that can be useful as a periodic monitoring tool and useful for scientific societies. *Conclusions*: The evolution of social robots represents an unstoppable process as does the increase in the aging of the population. Stakeholders must not look with suspicion toward these devices, which can represent an important resource, but rather invest in monitoring and consensus training initiatives.

Keywords: e-health; medical devices; m-health; rehabilitation; robotics; organization models; artificial intelligence; electronic surveys; social robots; collaborative robots

Citation: Simeoni, R.; Colonnelli, F.; Eutizi, V.; Marchetti, M.; Paolini, E.; Papalini, V.; Punturo, A.; Salvò, A.; Scipinotti, N.; Serpente, C.; et al. The Social Robot and the Digital Physiotherapist: Are We Ready for the Team Play? *Healthcare* **2021**, *9*, 1454. https://doi.org/10.3390/healthcare9111454

Academic Editor: Tin-Chih Toly Chen

Received: 12 August 2021
Accepted: 23 October 2021
Published: 27 October 2021

Publisher's Note: MDPI stays neutral with regard to jurisdictional claims in published maps and institutional affiliations.

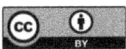

Copyright: © 2021 by the authors. Licensee MDPI, Basel, Switzerland. This article is an open access article distributed under the terms and conditions of the Creative Commons Attribution (CC BY) license (https://creativecommons.org/licenses/by/4.0/).

1. Introduction

Robotics has made it possible to introduce social robots (SRs) in both remote rehabilitation and assistance as a valid support in several sectors both as a direct and practical support and as a mediator [1–3]. The SR also stands as one of the key tools in rehabilitation through robotics as highlighted in the special issue Rehabilitation and Robotics: Are They Working Well Together? [4], of which this study aims to be a part.

It is natural that with this evolution, it is important to reflect on new professional figures or at least on the remodeling of already existing professional figures. One of the key figures in physical rehabilitation and assistance is that of the physiotherapist, who stands between the physician of physical medicine and rehabilitation and the patient, entering with greater contact with the patient. New models of care emerged, during the COVID-19 pandemic, based on technologies that allow greater social distancing between the patient and the therapist. Based on this, an expansion of the job description of many figures involved in rehabilitation and assistance is emerging. This is closely related to the remodeling of the *work-flow* that SRs have the potential to modify. Changes in the *work-flow* have a direct impact on the job description of the worker and therefore on the tasks he or she must perform, which are regulated by operational prescriptions in the workplace. Among the figures involved in this change and expansion of the job description, we find the figure of the physiotherapist. Regarding the figure of the physiotherapist, since the COVID-19 pandemic, it is preferred that when we mention a therapist with extended tasks toward digital in person or remotely (for example in remote therapy), we refer to the *augmented physiotherapist* (APT) or *digital physiotherapist* (DPT). This figure must be rethought starting from the new interaction tasks emerging in the COVID-19 era with the looming social distancing. Furthermore, the physical and rehabilitative medicine sector is moving in this direction. For some years now, there has been talk of new forms of therapy delivery in this area in virtual mode through remote digital communication or using new tools such as the SRs. For example, Alam Le has focused on this and analyzed the critical issues highlighted in the current pandemic and the previous pandemic experiences, analyzed the changes already requested by some key figures of the health system in relation to technologies due to new intervention models consolidated during the current epidemic, and reported some consensus studies on digital rehabilitation focused around the new figure of the *DPT* without forgetting the ethical and curricular aspects [5].

The SRs in their collaborative interaction have many capabilities: establishing and maintaining social relationships; learning social skills development and role models; using "natural" signals, such as gestures and gaze; expressing emotions as well as perceiving them; communicating with high-level dialogue; and expressing one's own personality and distinctive character. We can use SRs for a variety of purposes; for example, as educational tools and therapeutic aids [2,3]. There are several examples of SRs designed for use by elderly people [6–9] but also for frail and/or handicapped subjects needing rehabilitation and assistance: for example [10–15], to support certain motor activities; support during feeding; support during displacements; support them in drug therapy—for example, by reminding them to take a drug; support them from a cognitive point of view—for example, by stimulating them with games and supporting them from the point of view of communicative interaction, even as simple company; provide support as a hospital assistant; provide support as a mediator to therapists and/or relatives.

Furthermore, in the COVID-19 era, there has been an increase in the use of SRs in the above-listed desirable activities due to the necessary supervening obligation of social distancing to combat the pandemic [2]. The COVID-19 pandemic has created an unprecedented incentive for the development of the technologies in healthcare. This development involved both the boost and regulation of already consolidated solutions and the exploration of new potentials. All this certainly concerned digital health in the countless applications of *mHealth* and *eHealth*, but it also concerned other technologies, such as mechatronics applied in healthcare as in rehabilitation and assistance robotics [16]. Among the mechatronic devices that have had an important push in this period, we certainly find the SRs. If we focus on PubMed, we can immediately see how in 2020 (the year of the pandemic), we had 413 publications on SR, which was an increase of 24.8% compared to the number in 2019. In the first 4 months of 2021, furthermore, we already have 190 publications on SR, which is a trend that if confirmed by the end of the year could lead us to almost double the number of publications compared to those of 2019. As already highlighted for *mHealth* and *eHealth* technologies, it is particularly important to analyze the impact of innovative technologies on humans at work and in living environments. Regarding artificial intelligence, in a previous study, we analyzed the importance of the consent of digital radiology operators in view of a post-pandemic use through the proposition of targeted/calibrated surveys for those who will then have to work with technology [17]. In social robotics, the focus of this study, powerful efforts in algorithms are being made through artificial intelligence to allow continuous improvement of the SR in carrying out its role as an interaction with the human subject. A lot is expected of artificial intelligence (AI) in these devices. We expect the elimination or minimization of weaknesses of the mechatronic system such as the lack of empathy, of psychological perception, and of the capacity for discernment, which are all fundamental aspects if you want to position this device firmly in the role of collaborator and/or professional assistant. The AI is currently used to face this [18–25]: for example, to (a) help in recognizing facial expressions [18,19] and consequently propose adaptations; (b) improve aspects such as empathy [24,25]; (c) adapt the environments of life built around the individual [23]; (d) improve the acceptance and the prospects for the use of these technologies [20–22]. As in the studies proposed in [26,27], here too, we feel the need to investigate the consensus of the figures involved (physiotherapists) on the use of innovative AI-based devices that can radically change work patterns. Many figures are revolving around the SRs, ranging from the bioengineer to the physiotherapist without neglecting the stakeholders. One of the key figures regarding the interaction with the SR is that of the physiotherapist; therefore, the consensus of this figure around social robotics is strategic.

The purpose of the study was to investigate the consensus of the physiotherapists around the introduction of the SRs in the clinical practice both in rehabilitation and assistance. To achieve the main goal, we have decided to (a) develop a tool based on an *electronic survey* (eS) focused on the social robotics applied to the rehabilitation and assistance; and (b) submit the eS to physiotherapists to investigate their opinion and their level of consent on the topic. We have also decided to assess the acceptance of the eS on the physiotherapists who have participated in the study, in consideration of future uses in this area. An *electronic feedback form* (eFF) was designed for this.

The study is organized as follows.

Section Two (I) describes the methodology used in the technological choice, development, and administration of the electronic survey; it also (II) reports the inclusion protocol and study participants. *Section Three* reports (III) the output relating to the administration of the survey to the participants included in the study, divided by the types of application forms used (graded questions, Likert, and multiple choice), and (IV) the respondents' feedback on the electronic survey and employment prospects. *Section Four* discusses the evidence that emerged from the study and in particular, (V) the degree of consensus/acceptance on the introduction of the SR in healthcare and (VI) the high acceptance of the method, based on an electronic survey, as a periodic monitoring tool.

2. Materials and Methods

We have decided to develop the survey electronically; this allows both ease of administration using very convenient IT tools and ease of data collection. These tools have also the possibility of automatic reporting. Microsoft Forms was chosen in this study. It is available in the Microsoft 365 App Business Premium suite provided in the workplace. All users can access through their own domain account guaranteed by the corporate cybersecurity standards (which must comply with the international regulations in force) supported both by the *system security tools/system policy* and network *security*. The use of both an internal recommended tool (respecting the cybersecurity) and the plan to submit the *eS* anonymously simplified the authorization process (see the footnote).

We developed the sections of the eS with different types of questions: open question, choice, multiple choice, Likert, and graded questions. In the graded questions and the Likert, we fixed a six-level psychometric scale; therefore, it was possible to assign a minimum score of one and a maximum of six with a theoretical mean value (TMV) of 3.5. We can refer to the TMV for comparison in the analysis of the answers. An average value of the answers below TMV indicates *a more negative than positive response*. An average value above TMV indicates a *more positive than negative response*. In consideration of the objective of this study and the survey, we also managed the survey as a virtual focus group with careful considerations to the consensus issues related to all the aspects of the introduction of the SR. We started from the training up to the relationships between the SR in the several potential activities of involvement, with also the idea to create a stable product for the scientific societies. The study was designed at the Catholic University (CU) headquarters in Rome and San Martino al Cimino (Viterbo) and ran from 15 May 2021 to 15 July 2021. Regarding the address of the survey, we turned to physiotherapists under their course of the study (*PUCS*) and after the course of the study (*PACS*). We considered new graduates from less than a year to belong to the first group and those who then undertook a further specialization to belong to the second. The minimum age was 23 years; the maximum age was 58; Table 1 reports the demographic data.

Table 1. Characteristics of the participants in the two electronic-based submissions: the PUCS and the PACS.

Submission	Number Invited	Participants	Males/Females	Min Age/Max Age	Mean Age
Physiotherapists under the course of the study (PUCS)	161	156	79/77	23/35	24.3
Physiotherapists after the course of the study (PACS)	170	167	86/81	25/58	42.4

Therefore, we disseminated it with respect to the current regulations (see footnote at the end) using the mobile technology through social media, such as Facebook, LinkedIn, Twitter, Instagram, and WhatsApp; scientific and professional associations; and, in general, a *peer-to-peer* dissemination to collect data in the extended territory and therefore not limited to the CU.

We also submitted to all participants an electronic feedback form (*eFF*) based on the same technologies with a few questions of a graded evaluation type to investigate the acceptance of the eS in term of the robustness of the tool and to investigate the prospects.

We planned a dedicated post-processing analysis of the eS after submission.

The WEB link of the interactive tool eS is reported in [28]. The printout of the eS is reported in [29].

3. Results

The results are organized in two parts:
- Output of the survey administration.
- Output related to feedback on acceptance of the proposed electronic survey methodology and prospects.

3.1. The Outcome of the Electronic Survey

<u>The questionnaire in brief</u>

The questionnaire includes *25 questions*, as anticipated, of different types, including open questions, to have as broad a view as possible. *Questions 1–7* collect information about the informant (age, sex, training received, and membership in scientific societies). The *graded questions 8, 12–13,* and *19–20* are on the knowledge of SRs in general, on the impact in the world of assistance and physiotherapy, and on the influence of AI and ethics. *The questions through Likert modules 10, 14, and 15* address the detailed knowledge and the strengths and weaknesses perceived on the SRs. The *multiple-choice questions 16–18* address aspects related to the *workflow* changes and the relative role of the SR and physiotherapist. The remaining *questions 9, 21–25* accompany the others and/or are designed to indicate further wishes in this area.

First considerations

The age distribution of the two samples was normal, both when they were considered separately and jointly. Since the number of recruits exceeded 50 for each sample, the Kolmogorov–Smirnov test was chosen and preferred to Shapiro–Wilk [30–32]. To the question relating to knowledge in general, "*Q8. What is your level of knowledge of social robots in general?*", the PUCS group reported an average score of 3.83, while the PACS group reported an average score of 3.87. Student's *t*-test showed no significant differences ($p = 0.009$) [33].

The first analysis on the graded questions

The results in Table 2 show, for all the recruited, an average value above TMV (3.5) that indicates a more positive than negative response. Results show a high value in the answers to the questions:

- *Q12. How useful do you think the social robot can be in physiotherapy?*
- *Q13. How useful do you think the social robot can be in assistance?*

In addition, the answer to "*Q19. Do you think that the artificial intelligence will help improve this device by eliminating weaknesses?*" showed great confidence in artificial intelligence.

The participants consider ethics as an obstacle to the spread of the device, as evidenced by the high score given to the answer "*Q20. Do you think that issues relating to ethics will be an obstacle to the spread of this device?*

Table 2 shows that the percentage was never lower than 82.05%, which gave a value ≥ 4, with a high significance ($p < 0.01$, test $\chi 2$). For the two groups considered separately, the $\chi 2$ test reported the same significance ($p < 0.01$).

The second analysis on the Likert questions

The average values, for all the recruited, were above TMV (3.5) for all the Likert questions. This indicates a more positive than negative response for all three Likert questions:

- *Q10. Degree of knowledge on social robots?*
- *Q14. What are the strengths of social robots?*
- *Q15. What are the weaknesses of social robots?*

Table 2. Results relating to the graded questions with the details of the assessment.

Question	N(1)	N(2)	N(3)	N(4)	N(5)	N(6)	Mean
Q12. How useful do you think the social robot can be in physiotherapy?	9	17	8	98	102	89	4.65
Q13. How useful do you think the social robot can be in assistance?	10	8	2	52	115	136	5.04
Q19. Do you think that the artificial intelligence will help improve this device by eliminating weaknesses?	1	4	11	3	129	175	5.41
Q20. Do you think that issues relating to ethics will be an obstacle to the spread of this device?	9	1	8	7	87	211	5.46

Table 3 reports the most two popular questions for each Likert.

For Likert Q10, we had "*Robots for the elderly*" and "*Robots for people with communication disabilities*".

For Likert Q14, we had "*It does not judge*" and "*reliable*".

For Likert Q15, we had "*Lack of empathy*" and "*Risk of false relationships*".

Table 3. Results related to the two most popular answers of each Likert with the details of the assessment.

Likert/-Most Popular Answer-	N(1)	N(2)	N(3)	N(4)	N(5)	N(6)	Mean
Q.10. Degree of knowledge on social robots?/-Robots for the elderly-	12	9	14	27	85	176	5.14
Q.10. Degree of knowledge on social robots?/-Robots for people with communication disabilities-	14	13	16	28	84	168	5.04
Q.14. What are the strengths of social robots?/-It does not judge-	4	10	5	12	90	202	5.41
Q.14. What are the strengths of social robots?/-Reliable-	10	11	10	96	39	157	4.90
Q.15. What are the weaknesses of social robots?/-Lack of empathy-	9	12	7	27	87	181	5.21
Q.15. What are the weaknesses of social robots?/-Risk of false relationships-	7	12	10	97	37	160	4.93

Table 3 shows that the percentage was never lower than 86.69%, which gave a value ≥ 4, with a high significance ($p < 0.01$, test $\chi 2$). For the two groups considered separately, the $\chi 2$ test reported the same significance ($p < 0.01$).

The third analysis on the multiple choice questions

We report also for the multiple choice questions the two most popular answers. Table 4 shows the outcome.

Table 4. Feedback form output.

Question	N(1)	N(2)	N(3)	N(4)	N(5)	N(6)	Mean
Evaluate the survey as a tool for periodic monitoring and useful for the scientific societies	0	0	0	96	79	137	5.13
Evaluate the survey as a tool to obtain structured information from virtual focus groups	0	0	0	99	77	136	5.11
Evaluate the survey in general as a specific tool for the social robot	0	0	0	58	93	161	5.33
How user-friendly was the tool?	0	0	0	94	80	138	5.14
How effective was the tool	0	0	0	111	81	120	5.02
How complete was the tool?	0	0	0	74	89	149	5.24
How clear was the tool?	0	0	0	104	88	120	5.05
How functional was the tool?	0	0	0	103	74	135	5.10

For question Q9, "Where did you hear about it?", the most two popular statements were "Internet" (number of votes = 175) and "University" (number of votes = 168). The respondents also had the possibility of indicating "Other" among the answers. This possibility eventually allowed those who had had direct knowledge of the SRs in the field to make it explicit and detailed. No one has selected this field to indicate direct acquaintance. This is in line with the national situation where the use of these systems is still rare.

For question Q16, "I think in the future, the social robot . . . ", the most two popular statements were "It will be useful but complementary" (number of votes = 194) and "It will not catch on" (number of votes = 147).

Questions Q17 and Q18 are particularly strategic in consideration of the impact on the model of work in the field and on the revisiting of the job description (changing with the modifications of the workflow) of the future DPT and/or APT.

For question Q17, As a physiotherapist, how can I be useful to the social robot?, the most two popular statements were "As an operational manager of its use" (number of votes = 168) and "In performance monitoring" (number of votes = 155).

For question Q18, How will the social robot be useful to my profession?, the most two popular statements were "Increase in working capacity" (number of votes = 158) and "Facilitates integration with other professionals" (number of votes = 147).

3.2. The outcome of the Electronic Feedback Form

An important aspect of our survey is that relating to the opinion on the usefulness of the proposed questionnaire. A total of 312 out of 323 participants submitted feedback. Table 4 shows, on a six-value scale, the high acceptance of the methodology both in terms of the prospects of the survey in general (Questions 1–3) and some important characteristics taken into consideration (Questions 4–8). The table shows the following:

- All average ratings are above 5.0;
- No minimum rating is less than 4 (>TMV = 3.5), indicating that in all cases and for all questions, the instrument has always received a positive rating (more yes than no);
- The question "Evaluate the survey in general as a specific tool for the social robot" received the highest score, clearly indicating an important perspective for using the survey tool.

4. Discussion

The COVID-19 pandemic has created an unprecedented incentive for the development of the technologies in healthcare. This development involved both the boost and regulation of already consolidated solutions and the exploration of new potentials.

All this certainly concerned digital health in the countless applications of *mHealth* and *eHealth* but also other technologies, such as mechatronics applied in healthcare as in rehabilitation and assistance robotics [16]. Among the mechatronic devices that have had an important push in this period, we certainly find the SRs [1]. Many professional figures are revolving around the SR device, ranging from the bioengineer to the physiotherapist without neglecting the stakeholders (who in a rationalization of resources can also be economists). Among these figures, we find that for the physiotherapist, we are witnessing two phenomena. The first is that the physiotherapist is increasingly becoming a figure that has to do with *Digital Health*, so much so that today, we talk about an *augmented physiotherapist* (APT) and/or *digital physiotherapist* (DPT) [5]. On the other hand, the SRs through research are improving more and more in the aspects of social interaction thanks also to artificial intelligence [18–25].

It begins to become important or even strategic to investigate how SRs and physiotherapists are approaching and becoming familiar.

In this study, we have proposed a useful investigation, in view of consensus studies/conferences/guideline that can be used for the introduction of methods based on SRs in rehabilitation practices.

Therefore, we have developed an electronic survey focused on social robot-based rehabilitation and assistance and submitted it to physiotherapists in the field or in training to investigate their opinion and their level of consent regarding the use of the SR in rehabilitation and assistance. The outcome of the study has several polarities.

A *first polarity* consists of having designed a methodology based on the electronic surveys that allows the investigation of different aspects of the introduction of the SRs and on the relevant relationship with the figure of the DPT (or APT).

The *second polarity* consists on having verified by the physiotherapists the consensus/acceptance on the introduction of the SR in the healthcare. From the analysis of the subjects involved in the study, the following emerged in particular:

1. A coherent consensus and acceptance;
2. A high degree of knowledge of these systems;
3. The clear conviction on: (a) the usefulness of these systems in both rehabilitation and assistance; (b) that the artificial intelligence will be of aid in reducing the weakness of the device and (c) the ethical issues will hamper the use of this device;
4. A coherent vision on the strengths and the weakness of this device as highlighted in the Likert questions. In particular, among the strengths, the most voted were "It does not judge" and "It is reliable"; while among the weakness, the most voted were "The lack of empathy" and "The risk of false relationships".

The *third polarity* consists of having investigated, using multiple-choice questions, the vision strictly related to the evolution of their *job description* correlated to the changes of the *workflow* with the introduction of the SR. The physiotherapists are convinced that (a) they will be particularly useful with the SR both "*As an operational manager of its use*" and "*In performance monitoring*; (b) the SR will particularly aid them in the "*Increase in working capacity*" and "*Facilitating the integration with other professionals*".

The *fourth polarity* consists of an acceptance of feedback from the figures involved, in relation to the electronic tools of investigation proposed in the study. This feedback is useful for planning future initiatives and interventions.

From a general point of view, the study presents four added values.

The *first added value* is the product [28,29] represented by the electronic survey tool that can be easily submitted through the *mobile technologies* on the net during the pandemic. The *second added value* is represented by the survey with a wide range of aspects related to the use of the SRs and the direct impact on the *workflow* and therefore on the *job description* of the physiotherapist, having more and more to interact with the digital technologies in the pandemic era. The *third added value* is represented by the possibility of using this product, after minimal changes even in non-pandemic/post-pandemic periods for example by scientific and/or professional societies, to monitor as both a technological and social sensor the evolution of the topic. The *fourth added value* is represented by the outcome with reference to the two groups of *PUCS* and *PACS*, which is promptly useful for the stakeholders. The *fifth added value* lies in the outcome of the feedback form, which highlights how the tool has been appreciated both in terms of design and effectiveness of administration and how it is believed that it can be useful in the hands of scientific societies for periodic monitoring.

An important message emerges from the study for stakeholders. They must consider that the technological evolutions of SRs represent an unstoppable process, as well as the increase in the aging of the population [26,27]. They must not look with suspicion toward these devices, which can represent an important resource, but rather invest in monitoring and consensus training initiatives also through survey tools [17].This study certainly has the limitation of not having been able to administer a sweeping survey and on all professional figures, but it has the advantage of having proposed a useful, accepted automatic tool and the application of the survey methodology on a first sample that shows important evidence. From a general point of view, this article supports the initiatives that aim to facilitate the work of the physiotherapists when using the SRs with clear rules and a highly shared consensus. Future developments of the study foresee, after further targeted data-mining, an improvement of the electronic survey and a standardization of the same as a tool in the hands of scientific societies for periodic monitoring and investigations useful for making decisions and making improvements in the introduction of technology into the work routine.

5. Conclusions

SRs are bursting into health systems and playing a key role in many sectors, including rehabilitation [2]. The recent pandemic has accelerated this process [1]. It is foreseeable that in the coming years, many professionals in the health sector will have to deal with these devices through new working models based on SRs [26,27]. These systems involve and will involve figures who have to do with the elderly [6–9], frail, and handicapped individuals with motor and communication problems [10–15]. These systems involve and will involve figures who have to do with the elderly, frail, and handicapped individuals with motor and communication problems. Physiotherapists are certainly among the key figures, and recently, and in the pandemic period, they have had to deal more and more with digitization processes [5]. In this study, we focused on the figure of the physiotherapist, and we prepared a survey focused on the consensus and opinion of the use of this device. This study involved submitting an electronic survey on two statistically independent samples to collect and analyze the data automatically. The survey showed a consistency of the results on the investigated sample from which interesting considerations emerge.

Contrary to stereotypes that report how AI-based devices put jobs at risk; physiotherapists are not afraid of these devices. Physiotherapists believe that SRs can be reliable co-workers who do not judge. They believe that yes, SRs have weaknesses such as the lack of empathy and they risk creating false relationships, but they also believe that artificial intelligence on the one hand and wise professional use on the other will help overcome these limits. Physiotherapists also believe that SRs will remain a complementary tool and that their role will be of the utmost importance as an operational manager of its use and in performance monitoring. These professionals also believe that the device will allow an increase in working capacity and facilitate integration with other professionals.

All those involved in the study believe that the proposed electronic survey has proved to be a useful and effective tool that allows an *instantaneous creation of virtual focus groups*. They believe in this tool and believe that it can be useful as a periodic monitoring tool and useful for scientific societies.

Author Contributions: Data curation, All; Formal analysis, E.P., V.P., A.S., A.P., G.M., N.S., F.C. and D.G.; Funding acquisition, R.S., R.T. and D.G.; Investigation, R.T., C.S., V.E., M.M., E.P., V.P. and D.G.; Methodology, A.P., G.M., E.B. and D.G.; Resources, D.G.; Software, R.S., R.T., C.S. and D.G.; Supervision, D.G.; Visualization, R.S.; Writing—original draft, D.G.; Revision and approval of the manuscript, All. All authors have read and agreed to the published version of the manuscript.

Funding: This research received no external funding.

Institutional Review Board Statement: Not applicable. The study was conducted anonymously, and it has not included human or animal experimentation. The questionnaire is anonymous, and the topic did not concern clinical trials on humans but only opinions and expressions of their thoughts.

Informed Consent Statement: Not applicable.

Data Availability Statement: Not applicable.

Conflicts of Interest: The authors declare no conflict of interest.

References

1. Giansanti, D. The Social Robot in Rehabilitation and Assistance: What Is the Future? *Healthcare* **2021**, *9*, 244. [CrossRef] [PubMed]
2. Sheridan, T.B. A review of recent research in social robotics. *Curr. Opin. Psychol.* **2020**, *36*, 7–12. [CrossRef] [PubMed]
3. Atashzar, S.F.; Carriere, J.; Tavakoli, M. Review: How Can Intelligent Robots and Smart Mechatronic Modules Facilitate Remote Assessment, Assistance, and Rehabilitation for Isolated Adults With Neuro-Musculoskeletal Conditions? *Front. Robot. AI* **2021**, *8*, 610529. [CrossRef] [PubMed]
4. Giansanti, D. The Rehabilitation and the Robotics: Are They Going Together Well? *Health* **2020**, *9*, 26. [CrossRef]
5. Lee, A.C. COVID-19 and the Advancement of Digital Physical Therapist Practice and Telehealth. *Phys. Ther.* **2020**, *100*, 1054–1057. [CrossRef]
6. Ziaeetabar, F.; Pomp, J.; Pfeiffer, S.; El-Sourani, N.; Schubotz, R.I.; Tamosiunaite, M.; Wörgötter, F. Using enriched semantic event chains to model human action prediction based on (minimal) spatial information. *PLoS ONE* **2020**, *15*, e0243829. [CrossRef]
7. Hirt, J.; Ballhausen, N.; Hering, A.; Kliegel, M.; Beer, T.; Meyer, G. Social Robot Interventions for People with Dementia: A Systematic Review on Effects and Quality of Reporting. *J. Alzheimer's Dis.* **2021**, *79*, 773–792. [CrossRef]
8. Pu, L.; Moyle, W.; Jones, C.; Todorovic, M. The effect of a social robot intervention on sleep and motor activity of people living with dementia and chronic pain: A pilot randomized controlled trial. *Maturitas* **2021**, *144*, 16–22. [CrossRef]
9. Chen, K. Use of Gerontechnology to Assist Older Adults to Cope with the COVID-19 Pandemic. *J. Am. Med. Dir. Assoc.* **2020**, *21*, 983–984. [CrossRef]
10. Lewis, T.T.; Kim, H.; Darcy-Mahoney, A.; Waldron, M.; Lee, W.H.; Park, C.H. Robotic Uses in Pediatric Care: A Comprehensive Review. *J. Pediatr. Nurs.* **2021**, *58*, 65–75. [CrossRef]
11. Soares, E.E.; Bausback, K.; Beard, C.L.; Higinbotham, M.; Bunge, E.L.; Gengoux, G.W. Social Skills Training for Autism Spectrum Disorder: A Meta-analysis of In-person and Technological Interventions. *J. Technol. Behav. Sci.* **2021**, *6*, 166–180. [CrossRef]
12. Egido-García, V.; Estévez, D.; Corrales-Paredes, A.; Terrón-López, M.-J.; Velasco-Quintana, P.-J. Integration of a Social Robot in a Pedagogical and Logopedic Intervention with Children: A Case Study. *Sensors* **2020**, *20*, 6483. [CrossRef]
13. So, W.-C.; Cheng, C.-H.; Law, W.-W.; Wong, T.; Lee, C.; Kwok, F.-Y.; Lee, S.-H.; Lam, K.-Y. Robot dramas may improve joint attention of Chinese-speaking low-functioning children with autism: Stepped wedge trials. *Disabil. Rehabil. Assist. Technol.* **2020**, *2020*, 1841836. [CrossRef] [PubMed]

14. Sandgreen, H.; Frederiksen, L.H.; Bilenberg, N. Digital Interventions for Autism Spectrum Disorder: A Meta-analysis. *J. Autism Dev. Disord.* **2021**, *51*, 3138–3152. [CrossRef]
15. Pontikas, C.-M.; Tsoukalas, E.; Serdari, A. A map of assistive technology educative instruments in neurodevelopmental disorders. *Disabil. Rehabil. Assist. Technol.* **2020**, *30*, 1–9. [CrossRef] [PubMed]
16. Bartosiak, M.; Bonelli, G.; Maffioli, L.S.; Palaoro, U.; Dentali, F.; Poggialini, G.; Pagliarin, F.; Denicolai, S.; Previtali, P. Advanced Robotics as a Support in Healthcare Organizational Response. A COVID-19 Pandemic case. *Health Manag. Forum* **2021**. [CrossRef]
17. Salomon, J.A.; Reinhart, A.; Bilinski, A.; Chua, E.J.; La Motte-Kerr, W.; Rönn, M.; Reitsma, M.; Morris, K.A.; LaRocca, S.; Farag, T.; et al. The U.S. COVID-19 Trends and Impact Survey, 2020–2021: Continuous real-time measurement of COVID-19 symptoms, risks, protective behaviors, testing and vaccination. *MedRxiv* **2021**. [CrossRef]
18. Ramis, S.; Buades, J.M.; Perales, F.J. Using a Social Robot to Evaluate Facial Expressions in the Wild. *Sensors* **2020**, *20*, 6716. [CrossRef]
19. Song, Y.; Luximon, Y. Trust in AI Agent: A Systematic Review of Facial Anthropomorphic Trustworthiness for Social Robot Design. *Sensors* **2020**, *20*, 5087. [CrossRef]
20. Horstmann, A.C.; Krämer, N.C. Expectations vs. actual behavior of a social robot: An experimental investigation of the effects of a social robot's interaction skill level and its expected future role on people's evaluations. *PLoS ONE* **2020**, *15*, e0238133. [CrossRef]
21. Ke, C.; Lou, V.W.-Q.; Tan, K.C.-K.; Wai, M.Y.; Chan, L.L. Changes in technology acceptance among older people with dementia: The role of social robot engagement. *Int. J. Med. Inform.* **2020**, *141*, 104241. [CrossRef]
22. Cruz-Sandoval, D.; Favela, J. Incorporating Conversational Strategies in a Social Robot to Interact with People with Dementia. *Dement. Geriatr. Cogn. Disord.* **2019**, *47*, 140–148. [CrossRef]
23. Calderita, L.V.; Vega, A.; Barroso-Ramírez, S.; Bustos, P.; Núñez, P. Designing a Cyber-Physical System for Ambient Assisted Living: A Use-Case Analysis for Social Robot Navigation in Caregiving Centers. *Sensors* **2020**, *20*, 4005. [CrossRef]
24. Pepito, J.A.; Ito, H.; Betriana, F.; Tanioka, T.; Locsin, R.C. Intelligent humanoid robots expressing artificial humanlike empathy in nursing situations. *Nurs. Philos.* **2020**, *21*, e12318. [CrossRef] [PubMed]
25. Kerasidou, A. Artificial intelligence and the ongoing need for empathy, compassion and trust in healthcare. *Bull. World Health Organ.* **2020**, *98*, 245–250. [CrossRef]
26. Mejia, C.; Kajikawa, Y. Bibliometric Analysis of Social Robotics Research: Identifying Research Trends and Knowledgebase. *Appl. Sci.* **2017**, *7*, 1316. [CrossRef]
27. Available online: https://www.mordorintelligence.com/industry-reports/socialrobotsmarket (accessed on 17 June 2021).
28. Available online: https://forms.office.com/Pages/ResponsePage.aspx?id=_ccwzxZmYkutg7V0sn1ZEvPNtNci4kVMpoVUounzQ3tUQTNWWDhPM0k1RjRFR1lPTE8yVUVKMTNETC4u (accessed on 22 October 2021).
29. Available online: https://drive.google.com/drive/folders/1_KCaE_cd-hsTNaSHKJdxo21sHUDqU40K?usp=sharing (accessed on 22 October 2021).
30. Srivastava, M.; Hui, T. On assessing multivariate normality based on shapiro-wilk W statistic. *Stat. Probab. Lett.* **1987**, *5*, 15–18. [CrossRef]
31. Rahman, M. Estimating the box-cox transformation via shapiro-wilk w statistic. *Commun. Algebra* **1999**, *28*, 223–241. [CrossRef]
32. Schultz, B.; Schultz, A.; Pichlmayr, I.; Bender, R. Testing the Gaussianity of the Human EEG During Anesthesia. *Methods Inf. Med.* **1992**, *31*, 56–59. [CrossRef]
33. Surhone, L.M.; Tennoe, M.T.; Henssonow, S.F. (Eds.) *Student's T-Test: Student's T-Distribution, Probability Distribution, Normal Distribution, Probability, Statistics, Generalised Hyperbolic Distribution, Guinness Brewery, William Sealy Gosset*; Beta Script Publishing: Beau Bassin-Rose Hill, Mauritius, 2010.

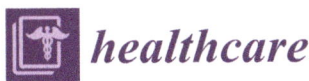

Article

The Effect of Early Applied Robot-Assisted Physiotherapy on Functional Independence Measure Score in Post-Myocardial Infarction Patients

Peter Bartík [1,*], Michal Vostrý [2,3,4], Zuzana Hudáková [5,6,7], Peter Šagát [1], Anna Lesňáková [5,7] and Andrej Dukát [8]

1. Health and Physical Education Department, Prince Sultan University, Riyadh 12435, Saudi Arabia; sagat@psu.edu.sa
2. Faculty of Education, J. E. Purkyně University, 40096 Ústí nad Labem, Czech Republic; michal.vostry@ujep.cz
3. Centre for Social Innovation and Inclusion in Education, J. E. Purkyně University, 40096 Ústí nad Labem, Czech Republic
4. Faculty of Medical Studies, J. E. Purkyně University, 40096 Ústí nad Labem, Czech Republic
5. Faculty of Health, Catholic University, 034 01 Ružomberok, Slovakia; zuzana.hudakova@ku.sk (Z.H.); anna.lesnakova@ku.sk (A.L.)
6. Department of Health Care Studies, College of Polytechnics, 58601 Jihlava, Czech Republic
7. SNP Central Military Hospital, Faculty Hospital, 034 01 Ružomberok, Slovakia
8. Fifth Department of Internal Medicine, Comenius University in Bratislava, 814 99 Bratislava, Slovakia; andrej.dukat@fmed.uniba.sk
* Correspondence: peter.bartik@post.sk; Tel.: +966-538546822

Abstract: Robot-assisted training has been widely used in rehabilitation programs, but no significant clinical evidence about its use in productive working-age cardiac patients was demonstrated. Thus, we hypothesized that early applied robot-assisted physiotherapy might provide additional treatment benefits in the rehabilitation of post-myocardial infarction (MI) patients. A total of 92 (50 men, 42 women) hospitalized post-MI patients with the age of 60.9 ± 2.32 participated in the research. An early intensive physiotherapy program ($7\times$/week, $2\times$/day) was applied for each patient with an average time of 45 min per session. Patients were consecutively assigned to Experimental group (EG) and Control group (CG). Then, 20 min of robot-assisted training by Motomed letto 2 or Thera-Trainer tigo was included in all EG physiotherapy sessions. The Functional Independence Measures (FIM) score at the admission and after 14 days of rehabilitation was used for an assessment. When analyzing time * group effect by repeated-measures ANOVA, we reported that EG showed a higher effect in ADL ($p = 0.00$), and Motor indicators ($p = 0.00$). There was no statistically significant effect reported in the Social indicator ($p = 0.35$). Early rehabilitation programs for post-MI patients might be enhanced by robotic tools, such as THERA-Trainer tigo, and Motomed letto 2. The improvement was particularly noticeable in mobility and ADLs.

Keywords: robot-assisted therapy; FIM score; myocardial infarction; first phase cardiac physiotherapy

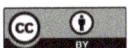

Citation: Bartík, P.; Vostrý, M.; Hudáková, Z.; Šagát, P.; Lesňáková, A.; Dukát, A. The Effect of Early Applied Robot-Assisted Physiotherapy on Functional Independence Measure Score in Post-Myocardial Infarction Patients. *Healthcare* 2022, 10, 937. https://doi.org/10.3390/healthcare10050937

Academic Editor: Daniele Giansanti

Received: 21 March 2022
Accepted: 16 May 2022
Published: 18 May 2022

Publisher's Note: MDPI stays neutral with regard to jurisdictional claims in published maps and institutional affiliations.

Copyright: © 2022 by the authors. Licensee MDPI, Basel, Switzerland. This article is an open access article distributed under the terms and conditions of the Creative Commons Attribution (CC BY) license (https://creativecommons.org/licenses/by/4.0/).

1. Introduction

Coronary heart disease (CHD) is the leading cause of morbidity and mortality worldwide. The most common form of CHD is myocardial infarction [1]. The number of post-MI patients hospitalized is increasing gradually. The basic therapeutic principles for the treatment of this disease are the same for all age groups. However, it is necessary to modify the treatment and subsequent therapy with respect to the patient's age [2]. Age is one of the decisive factors that has a major impact on the therapeutical process [3]. Other factors include gender and patients' individual needs. The therapy prescribed should take all these factors into account [4]. The incidence of MI increases with age. In the United States, people over 65 years represent 13% of the total population, but they form almost half of all hospitalized patients with this diagnosis. The MI prevalence in the population of 40–59 age is 3.3% in men, and 1.8% in women, while in the population of 60–79 age it is 11.3% in men, and 4.2% in women [5]. The incidence in the population of the Czech Republic is very similar, with the highest incidence rate in men and women in the 70 to 79 years age group [6]. In South Asians, the incidence is even higher in the most age groups. The incidence rate ratio is 1.45 for South Asian compared to non-South Asian men and 1.80 for South Asian women [7]. Based on the above stated, it is also important to note that elderly patients have a higher incidence of co-morbidities which may contribute to higher mortality [8]. In younger MI patients, positive family history is often present, while older patients suffer from hypertension, diabetes mellitus, or obesity more frequently [9]. The myocardial infarction is often atypical in diabetic patients. It is without common stenocardia, which is the reason why such patients seek medical attention only after developed complications have manifested [10].

The number of hospitalized post-MI patients is extensive, so it is a demand for effective rehabilitation. The target group in our study were patients of the active working age (<64 years) with a need for an effective physiotherapy process to be able to get back to the working process and daily life as soon as possible. The rehabilitation process of cardiac patients is divided into four phases. The first phase is focused on hospital rehabilitation and was the period of our investigation. Its main goal is to prevent deconditioning, thromboembolic complications, and to prepare the patient for discharge and return to normal daily life as soon as possible. The second phase is focused on immediate post-hospital rehabilitation. The duration is about three months and the focus is mainly on lifestyle change and adherence to secondary prevention. The third phase is a period of stabilization, in which the emphasis is on regular endurance training and consolidating changes in a healthy lifestyle. The last fourth phase is then focused on maintaining the status quo, which means regular, long-term compliance with said principles [11,12]. Despite the availability of the presented therapeutic options nowadays, it is important to mention the prognosis of the disease itself. It is worse in older patients than in the younger population. Improving the rehabilitation care of patients with myocardial infarction leads to a prolongation of their lives [13].

The current modern approach in inpatient rehabilitation is focused on robot-assisted therapy with regard to the body weight of patients which might be a limitation for rehabilitation procedures [14]. Robotic devices in rehabilitation we can see in use today are continuously under intensive development to improve their effectiveness in physiotherapy programs. In the case of traditional concepts of physiotherapy, it is directed mainly to achieving functional improvement of motor or cognitive abilities [15]. In the case of cardiac patients, robot-assisted training has been widely used in rehabilitation programs, but no significant clinical evidence to use it in productive working-age cardiac patients was demonstrated. Thus, the main contribution of this study is to provide the evidence supporting the usage of robotic tools in early rehabilitation stage of post-MI patients. We hypothesized that early applied robot-assisted physiotherapy might provide additional treatment benefits in the rehabilitation of post-MI patients. The purpose of the study was to investigate what is the effectiveness of robot-assisted physiotherapy in early stage post-MI patients of productive working age.

2. Materials and Methods

2.1. Subjects and Experimental Setup

The research sample consisted of 92 participants of the productive working-age 60.9 ± 2.32 (55–64 years), with a BMI of 32.2 ± 4.84, representing 50 men and 42 women. Data collection took place in the Department of cardiology, Masaryk Hospital, Ústí nad Labem, Czech Republic. All patients included in the study were hospitalized due to the myocardial infarction (MI), ICD codes—10: I21. The secondary diagnosis was obesity or diabetes mellitus, or a combination of both. All underwent early mobilization within the

2nd–3rd day of hospitalization after approval from a cardiologist. These patients were sufficiently stable to start cardiac rehabilitation based on the following conditions: stable blood pressure, stable heart rate (HR), no angina pectoris, no shortness of breath, Ejection fraction > 0.45, no resting or stress ischemia, and no arrhythmia. The following parameters were regularly assessed when in the physiotherapy sessions: Borg score below 13 (6–20), resting HR increased max + 20 bpm, HR below 120 bpm, exercise up to tolerance if non-symptomatic. If any parameter was not met, the training was completed only supine on the bed, or not at all if the symptoms persisted. Patients with complications were excluded from the research.

All patients had to pass the inclusion criteria. Data collection was performed consecutively. The first 46 patients (25 ♂/21 ♀) that passed the inclusion criteria formed the EG and the second 46 patients formed the CG. The original target of EG was a minimum of 50 (25 ♂/25 ♀). However, we reduced it by four on the female side due to the inability to recruit an appropriate number till the end of the time period devoted to the EG collection (one year). Afterward, the CG was formed (25 ♂/21 ♀) with the same inclusion criteria. The timeframe of the study lasted two years. The distribution of the subjects based on gender was equal in both research groups. We outline the whole process in the research flowchart (Figure 1). All patients that participated in the experiment were explained the research details before they signed the written consent. The participants were blinded to the research hypothesis.

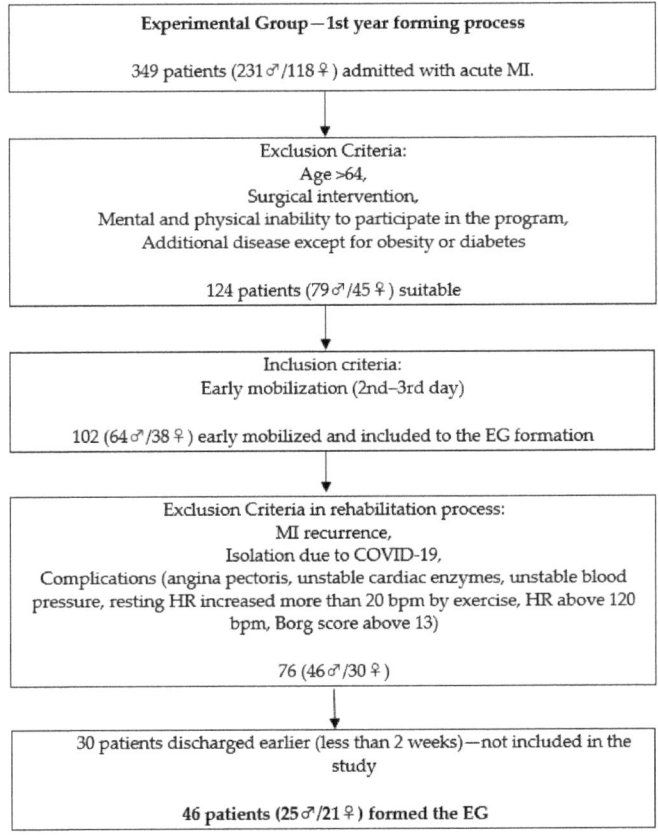

Figure 1. *Cont.*

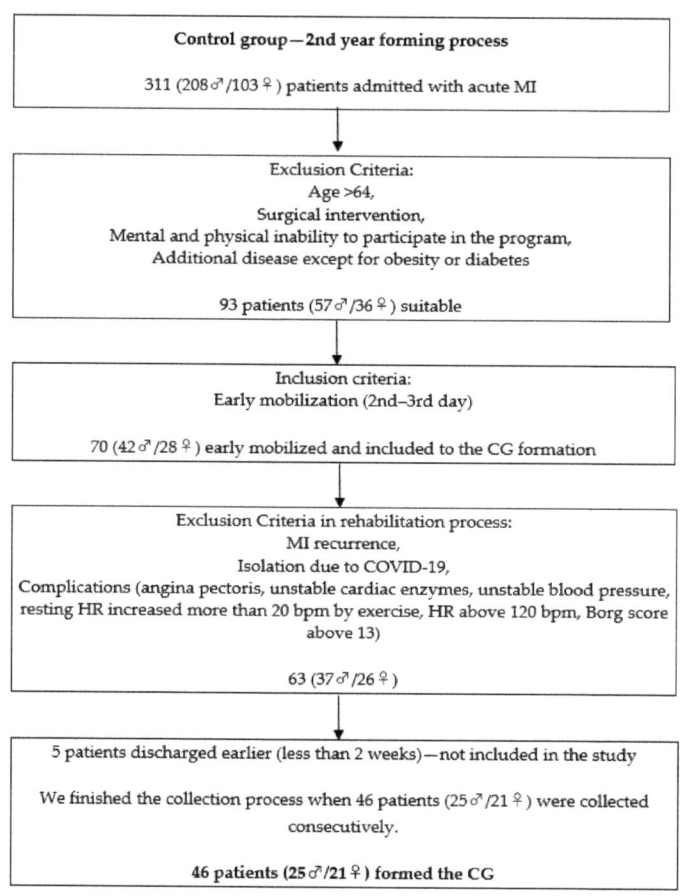

Figure 1. Research flowchart.

Inclusion criteria:
- Individuals after MI, ICD codes—10: I21;
- Age < 64;
- At least 1 days of physiotherapy training before discharge;
- Mental and physical ability to participate in the program;
- No active angina pectoris, stable cardiac enzymes, stable blood pressure, pulse, and respiratory rate within a range that allowed the patient to exercise;
- Early mobilization (2nd–3rd day of hospitalization);
- No surgical intervention (catheterization not included).
- Exclusion criteria:
- Early discharge from the unit (less than 14 days of physiotherapy program);
- Complicated recovery;
- MI recurrence;
- Late mobilization (more than third day);
- Additional disease except for obesity or diabetes;
- Isolation due to COVID-19.

2.2. Intervention

Both EG and CG participants started an early intensive physiotherapy program seven times a week (two times a day) with an average time of 45 min per session. The early program for patients after MI was focused on preventing decondition and thromboembolic complications, improving adaptation to physical activity, and preparing patients to return to ADLs. The early physiotherapy program was performed by four physiotherapists experienced in the field. The motivation factor was the same for both research groups since the study was blinded to the hospital staff. The type and intensity of exercise and the position (standing, sitting, lying in a supine position) depended on the patient's condition. Exercises in both EG and CG were the same except for the robotic intervention. The majority of movements performed during the physiotherapy sessions had repetitive analytical character, meaning they had the same range of motion and direction while it was not based on real-world situational biomechanics, such as functional movements. The movements were repetitively performed with specific phases and rhythm equal for both EG and CG.

Physiotherapy units for EG included active-assisted and active repetitive analytical movements of the upper and lower limbs lying on the bed (5 min), active exercise of repetitive analytical movements in a sitting position (5 min), mobilization to a standing position, and a short walk, active exercise of repetitive analytical movements in a standing position, and a short walk up and down the stairs (15 min). Then, 20 min of robot-assisted training with repetitive movements was implemented in all EG physiotherapy sessions. Both legs and arms were evenly involved in the training on a regular basis. Robotic device applications in EG always came with the start of the mobilization and rehabilitation program.

Physiotherapy units for CG included active-assisted and active repetitive analytical movements of the upper and lower limbs lying on the bed (10 min), active exercise of repetitive analytical movements in a sitting position (10 min), mobilization to a standing position, and a short walk, active exercise of repetitive analytical movements in a standing position, and a short walk up and down the stairs (25 min).

We applied the following devices for the early-stage rehabilitation program in EG: MOTOmed letto 2 (RECK-Technik GmbH & Co. KG, Betzenweiler, Germany), and THERA-Trainer tigo (Medizintechnik GmbH, Hochdorf, Germany).

MOTOmed letto 2 is a motor-assisted bed model training device with an automatic system for either legs or arms mobilization and training in a supine or sitting position often used for bed-ridden patients. THERA-Trainer tigo is a motor-assisted training device with an automatic system for either legs or arms mobilization, and training in a sitting position. Both devices allow passive, active-assisted, active, or active against resistance movements. The advantage of both is the possibility of application with the function of presetting and memory of training regime level. It is safe to let patients work out without active supervision. The presence of a physiotherapist is needed only at the beginning and the end of the training unit and when adjusting between arms and legs program. The position (supine or sitting), and the level of resistance for each EG patient was based on the actual condition. The training process had a tendency to increase the difficulty level of each following session, while the time was fixed from the beginning.

Both devices are regularly used in rehabilitation programs in our department, and their application is justified by several studies. Following authors reported a positive effect of MOTOMED letto 2 in the early physiotherapeutic intervention [16,17], while the positive effect of THERA-Trainer tigo was declared by the following researchers [18,19].

2.3. Assessment

The Functional Independence Measure (FIM) score is the standardized tool to evaluate the patient's functional level and independence on admission and discharge from the hospital. FIM score at the admission and after 14 days of rehabilitation (28 sessions) was used for an assessment of the subjects. Three indicators of FIM were evaluated individually—ADL, Motor, and Social. Standardized FIM record sheets in the Czech language were used.

All FIM scores were evaluated by four experienced physiotherapists working in the department. Both input and output assessments of the particular patient were always performed by the same physiotherapist. All physiotherapists included in the assessment and therapy process were blinded to the study details. We concluded the inter-rater reliability sufficient since it was performed by four trained and experienced physiotherapists and it is supported by scientific literature [20]. Orders for the specific physiotherapy interventions for CG and EG came only from the researcher working in the department after consultation with the cardiologist. The same researcher was regularly supervising the experiment process. However, he did not interfere with the FIM evaluation process.

Each item of the FIM (total score 18–126) is assessed by 1–7 points. Three research indicators are as follows:

ADL (score 8–56) includes eight items: eating, grooming, bathing, dressing the upper body, dressing lower body, toileting, bladder management, and bowel management;

MOTOR (score 5–35) includes five items: transfers—bed/chair/wheelchair, transfers—toilet, transfers—bath/shower, walk/wheelchair, stairs;

SOCIAL (score 5–35) includes five items: comprehension, expression, social interaction, problem solving, and memory [21].

2.4. Sample Size and Statistical Analysis

The sample size calculation was analyzed by the G*Power software version 3.1.9.4. The interval of confidence was set to 95%, the margin of error to 5%, and the probability of success to 0.5. It was determined that the minimum total sample size that should participate in the study to have a representative sample of the studied population was 54.

All data were analyzed using IBM SPSS version 25. Statistical analysis included a descriptive analysis of general characteristics by using the mean and standard deviation. Gender independence was analyzed by the Chi-square test. Normality of dataset distribution was analyzed by Kolmogorov–Smirnov and Shapiro–Wilk tests. The Paired T-test was used for the analysis of the FIM indicators differences. The Mann–Whitney U test was used for age, BMI, diabetes type II, Borg score, and HR differences comparisons. The time * group effect was analyzed using Repeated Measures ANOVA, taking the group as between factor and time as within factor. To estimate the effect size (ES), after applying the T-test in FIM indicators, the following formula was used: $ES = (X_1 - X_2)/\sqrt{(S_1^2 + S_2^2)/2}$. An ES of 0.2 was considered small, 0.5 moderate, and 0.8 large. The statistical significance threshold was set to 0.05.

3. Results

Data from 92 participants (50 male/42 female) of the productive working-age 60.9 ± 2.32 (55–64 years), with a BMI of 32.2 ± 4.84, were collected and included in the study. Table 1 reports the demographic characteristics, type II diabetes duration (years), maximum Borg score, resting HR, and maximum HR in effort of all participants, and between research groups differences. Borg score and HR data were obtained during the first day of the physiotherapy program and after one week. No statistically significant differences were reported between CG and EG. Table 2 reports FIM differences between the Admission and 14 days of rehabilitation, with the effect size (Cohen's d using pooled variance). Table 3 reports time * group analyses of three FIM indicators.

Table 1. Characteristics of participants.

Characteristic	CG	EG	Sig. (p-Value)
N (Male/Female)	46 (25/21)	46 (25/21)	-
Age (60.9 ± 2.32)	60.8 ± 2.56	60.9 ± 2.08	0.96
BMI (32.2 ± 4.84)	31.8 ± 5.04	32.7 ± 4.63	0.21
Diabetes duration (7.3 ± 3.48)	7.1 ± 2.99	7.5 ± 3.93	0.63
1st day of rehabilitation program			
Borg score (10.3 ± 1.76)	10.5 ± 1.50	10.1 ± 1.97	0.38
HR—rest (76.2 ± 8.29)	77.7 ± 8.71	74.7 ± 7.66	0.14
HR—effort (95.0 ± 5.80)	96.0 ± 5.49	93.9 ± 5.97	0.10
7th day of the rehabilitation program			
Borg score (10.5 ± 1.67)	10.46 ± 1.70	10.59 ± 1.65	0.73
HR—rest (75.0 ± 7.73)	75.8 ± 7.64	74.15 ± 7.81	0.34
HR—effort (96.5 ± 5.60)	97.2 ± 5.11	95.9 ± 6.05	0.13

CG—control group, EG—experimental group, BMI—body mass index, HR—heart rate, Sig.—significance.

Table 2. FIM differences between the admission and 14 days of rehabilitation.

FIM Category	Admission	14 Days of Rehabilitation	Difference	Cohen's d	Admission/14 Days of Rehabilitation Sig. (p-Value)
ADL (8–56)					
CG	45.11 ± 3.29	48.11 ± 3.99	2.98 ± 2.24	0.82	0.00
EG	45.67 ± 3.91	50.67 ± 3.49	5.02 ± 2.82	1.36	0.00
MOTOR (5–35)					
CG	16.52 ± 1.07	18.70 ± 1.44	2.17 ± 0.93	1.71	0.00
EG	16.61 ± 1.45	20.09 ± 1.63	3.48 ± 1.09	2.25	0.00
SOCIAL (5–35)					
CG	30.09 ± 2.31	31.38 ± 1.96	1.28 ± 1.36	0.60	0.00
EG	30.02 ± 2.22	31.07 ± 2.21	1.04 ± 1.03	0.47	0.00
TOTAL SCORE (18–126)					
CG	91.72 ± 4.65	98.17 ± 4.82	6.46 ± 3.17	1.36	0.00
EG	92.30 ± 5.07	101.83 ± 4.91	9.52 ± 3.06	1.91	0.00

FIM—functional independence measure, ADL—activities of daily living, CG—control group, EG—experimental group, Sd—standard deviation, Sig.—significance.

Table 3. Time * group analysis of FIM indicators.

FIM Category	Type III Sum of Squares	df	Mean Square	F	Sig. (p-Value)
ADL					
Time * Group	46.00	1	46.00	13.99	**0.00 ***
Motor					
Time * Group	19.57	1	19.57	38.24	**0.00 ***
Social					
Time * Group	0.66	1	0.66	0.90	**0.35**

FIM—functional independence measure, ADL—activities of daily living, df—degrees of freedom, F—variation between sample means, Sig.—significance.

The research brought the following findings. Standardized FIM Scores for both research groups at the admission ranged from Level 4 (Moderate assistance 72–89) to Level 5 (Supervision needed 90–107), and after 14 days of physiotherapy program from Level 5 to Level 6 (Modified independence 108–119). Patients of both groups improved significantly in two weeks in all three FIM indicators—ADL, Motor, and Social ($p < 0.05$).

When analyzing the time * group effect, we reported a statistically significant difference in the FIM-ADL indicator ($p = 0.00$), and the FIM-MOTOR indicator ($p = 0.00$). The effect of the therapy was higher in EG, where the robot-assisted intervention was included in the physiotherapy program. We did not report any statistically significant difference between groups in the FIM-SOCIAL indicator ($p = 0.35$).

4. Discussion

Our study revealed that early applied robot-assisted physiotherapy provided additional treatment benefits in the rehabilitation of post-MI patients. The Motomed letto 2 and Thera-Trainer tigo were used in our experiment. We reported a significant difference when analyzing the time * group effect of EG and CG by FIM results, particularly the FIM-ADL indicator, and the FIM-MOTOR indicator, while in the case of the FIM-SOCIAL indicator, we did not report any significant effect of the experimental therapy when time * group effect was evaluated. The presented results indicate an improvement in performing activities of daily living and mobility. The research group of patients improved mainly in the areas of verticalization, hygiene, and mobility. Taking into account an improvement in the monitored areas of the selected patients after two weeks of intervention, in general, we evaluate the combined robot-assisted therapy in a positive way. The robot-assisted rehabilitation effect is relatively unknown in the professional public when considering post-MI cardiac patients. No research has been published regarding this topic. There are studies confirming the positive effects of robot-assisted physiotherapy in research samples different from working-age post-MI cardiac patients presented in this study [22–25]. The above-mentioned authors reported additional treatment benefits when robotic physiotherapy was applied, while other studies are relatively skeptical of such claims putting it on the same level as the conventional approach with no extra benefits [26–28]. The other study concludes that although robot-assisted therapy can improve the motor skills of individuals, this phenomenon is not completely proven and further research is needed [29]. The presented results report that robot-assisted therapy might have a positive effect and bring additional treatment benefits to patients after myocardial infarction. The FIM indicators scores of the experimental group with robot-assisted physiotherapy intervention improved in ADLs and mobility with a statistically significant difference comparing the group with a casual physiotherapy approach. Based on the results we can recommend using robot-assisted devices in the early rehabilitation plan of post-MI patients. Robot-assisted physiotherapy has a tendency to be widely applied in the field even more in the following years considering the population aging trend which causes a need to adapt to the newly emerging demographic situation. The aim of such adaptation is primarily to prevent the exclusion and discrimination of the older age group where robot-assisted therapy might be very useful and effective. All interventions should lead to an active movement even during aging [2].

In recent years, robotic systems have been playing an increasingly important role in physiotherapy. The aim of these platforms is to aid the recovery process by assisting patients to perform a number of controlled tasks, thus effectively complementing the role of the physiotherapist [30]. The advantages of using modern devices in rehabilitation can be seen in many areas of human performance nowadays. A common feature of gait training robots is the possibility to support (partially or totally) the body weight and the movement of patients [31]. Mobile anthropomorphic robots are examples of such modern machines which assist in the operation of human muscles and are called exoskeletons [32,33].

Furthermore, movement therapy should be stimulated by the help of psychomotor therapy, special educational methods, and therapeutic physical education that must be intentionally applied and distributed. It is a supportive method that is in parallel with pharmacotherapy and surgical approach [34,35]. This intervention supports active movement together with elements of cognitive rehabilitation and training in performing activities of daily living. Finally, we would also like to point out that it is important to motivate patients for regular exercise, whether classic or robotic because it is the lack of motivation that can lead to negative results. The reason can often be a lack of interest or non-appreciation of the regular exercise results [36]. It is an important task for physiotherapists to motivate patients towards progress.

This research has its limitation as well. We understand that in these kind of data collection there is no absolute control of the relevant variables due to the lack of randomization, so it is more vulnerable to bias. Since this is only the first study exploring the robot-assisted therapy effect in the first phase of cardiac rehabilitation in post-MI patients, the other studies should follow. Our main objective was to assess the effect by FIM score, so the other methods of evaluation are recommended for future studies as well.

5. Conclusions

Early rehabilitation programs for post-myocardial infarction patients might be enhanced by robotic tools such as Thera-Trainer tigo, and MOTOmed letto 2. The improvement was particularly noticeable in the case of ADLs and motor abilities, supporting the application of early robot-assisted physiotherapy. This study is the first one investigating the early impact on cardiac post-IM patients.

Author Contributions: Conceptualization, P.B., M.V., P.Š.; methodology, P.B., M.V., A.D.; software, P.Š., Z.H., A.L.; validation, M.V., Z.H.; formal analysis, P.B.; investigation, M.V., Z.H., A.L.; resources, M.V., P.Š.; data curation, M.V., P.Š.; writing—original draft preparation, P.B., M.V.; writing—review and editing, P.B., M.V., Z.H., P.Š., A.L.; supervision, A.D.; All authors have read and agreed to the published version of the manuscript.

Funding: The authors would like to acknowledge the support of Prince Sultan University for paying the Article Processing Charges (APC) of this publication.

Institutional Review Board Statement: The study was conducted according to the guidelines of the Declaration of Helsinki and approved by the Institutional Review Board of Prince Sultan University, Riyadh, Saudi Arabia (protocol code PSU IRB-2021-10-0092).

Informed Consent Statement: Informed consent was obtained from all subjects involved in the study.

Data Availability Statement: The data presented in this study are available upon request from the corresponding author.

Conflicts of Interest: The authors declare no conflict of interest.

References

1. Jayaraj, J.C.; Davatyan, K.; Subramanian, S.S.; Priya, J. Epidemiology of myocardial infarction. *Myocard. Infarct.* **2019**, *3*, 10. [CrossRef]
2. Fischerová, B. Specifika akutního infarktu myokardu ve stáří. *Interní Med. Pro Praxi.* **2008**, *10*, 110–112.
3. Mumthas, A.; Abraham Varghese, V. Arrhythmia pattern in patients with acute myocardial infarction. *IAIM* **2019**, *6*, 142–148.
4. Rosengren, A.; Wallentin, L.; Simoons, M.; Gitt, A.K.; Behar, S.; Battler, A.; Hasdai, D. Age, clinical presentation, and outcome of acute coronary syndromes in the Euroheart acute coronary syndrome survey. *Eur. Heart J.* **2006**, *27*, 789–795. [CrossRef] [PubMed]
5. Mozaffarian, D.; Benjamin, E.J.; Go, A.S.; Arnett, D.K.; Blaha, M.J.; Cushman, M.; de Ferranti, S.; Després, J.P.; Fullerton, H.J.; Howard, V.J.; et al. American Heart Association Statistics Committee and Stroke Statistics Subcommittee. Heart disease and stroke statistics—2015 update: A report from the American Heart Association. *Circulation* **2015**, *131*, e29–e322. [CrossRef] [PubMed]
6. Dostál, O.; Bělohlávek, J.; Kovárník, P. Infarkt myokardu u starších pacientů. *Kardiol. Rev.* **2007**, *9*, 82–88.
7. Fischbacher, C.M.; Bhopal, R.; Povey, C.; Steiner, M.; Chalmers, J.; Mueller, G.; Jamieson, J.; Knowles, D. Record linked retrospective cohort study of 4.6 million people exploring ethnic variations in disease: Myocardial infarction in South Asians. *BMC Public Health* **2007**, *7*, 142. [CrossRef]
8. Berger, A.K.; Schulman, K.A.; Gersh, B.J.; Pirzada, S.; Breall, J.A.; Johnson, A.E.; Every, N.R. Primary coronary angioplasty vs thrombolysis for the management of acute myocardial infarction in elderly patients. *Jama* **1999**, *28*, 341–348. [CrossRef]
9. Clark, A.M.; King-Shier, K.M.; Thompson, D.R.; Spaling, M.A.; Duncan, A.S.; Stone, J.A.; Jaglal, S.B.; Angus, J.E. A qualitative systematic review of influences on attendance at cardiac rehabilitation programs after referral. *Am. Heart J.* **2012**, *164*, 835–845. [CrossRef]
10. Dietz, V. Body weight supported gait training: From laboratory to clinical setting. *Brain Res. Bull.* **2008**, *30*, 459–463. [CrossRef]
11. Chaloupka, V. Rehabilitace nemocných po infarktu myokardu. *Interní Med. Pro Praxi* **2005**, *6*, 74–78.
12. Želízko, M. Akutní infarkt myokardu s elevacemi ST úseku: Realita-výsledky registru NRKI (Sjezd ČKS 2007). In Proceedings of the XV Annual Congress of Czech Cardiologic Society, Brno, Czech Republic, 13–16 May 2007.
13. Špinar, J.; Vítovec, J. *Jak dobře žít s nemocným srdcem*; Grada: Praha, Czech Republic, 2007; ISBN 978-80-247-1822-4.
14. Mocan, M.; Mocan, B. Cardiac rehabilitation for older patients with cardiovascular pathology using robotic systems—A survey. *Balneo Res. J.* **2019**, *10*, 33–36. [CrossRef]
15. Siverová, J.; Bužgová, R. Reminiscence v péči o seniory s demencí. *Česká a Slovenská Psychiatrie* **2016**, *112*. Available online: https://scholar.google.com/scholar?hl=en&as_sdt=0%2C5&q=Siverov%C3%A1%2C+J.%3B+Bu%C5%BEgov%C3%A1%2C+R.+Reminiscence+v+p%C3%A9%C4%8Di+o+seniory+s+demenc%C3%AD&btnG= (accessed on 20 March 2022).

16. Prokazova, P.R.; Piradov, M.A.; Ryabinkina, Y.V.; Kunzevich, G.I.; Gnedovskaya, E.V.; Popova, L.A. Robot-assisted therapy using the MOTOmed letto 2 for the integrated early rehabilitation of stroke patients admitted to the intensive care unit. *Hum. Physiol.* **2016**, *42*, 885–890. [CrossRef]
17. De Beer, C.R.; Van Rooijen, A.J.; Pretorius, J.P.; Rheeder, P.; Becker, P.J.; Paruk, F. Muscle strength and endurance to predict successful extubation in mechanically ventilated patients: A pilot study evaluating the utility of upper-limb muscle strength and ergometry. *S. Afr. J. Crit. Care* **2018**, *34*, 44–49. [CrossRef]
18. Ramírez, J.J.L.; García, E.D.; Valladares, Y.C.; García, M.A.F.; Capetillo, N.A.M.; Martínez, V.M.V. Eficacia del Thera Trainer Tigo 510 en el tratamiento rehabilitador de niños con parálisis cerebral. *Revista Cubana de Medicina Física y Rehabilitación* **2021**, *13*, 1–16.
19. Meyer, S.; Verheyden, G.; Kempeneers, K.; Michielsen, M. Arm-hand boost therapy during inpatient stroke rehabilitation: A pilot randomized controlled trial. *Front. Neurol.* **2021**, *12*, 247. [CrossRef]
20. Hamilton, B.B.; Laughlin, J.A.; Fiedler, R.C.; Granger, C.V. Interrater reliability of the 7-level functional independence measure (FIM). *Scand. J. Rehabil. Med.* **1994**, *26*, 115–119.
21. Linacre, J.M.; Heinemann, A.W.; Wright, B.D.; Granger, C.V.; Hamilton, B.B. The structure and stability of the Functional Independence Measure. *Arch. Phys. Med. Rehabil.* **1994**, *75*, 127–132. [CrossRef]
22. Ammann-Reiffer, C.; Bastiaenen, C.H.; Meyer-Heim, A.D.; van Hedel, H.J. Effectiveness of robot-assisted gait training in children with cerebral palsy: A bicenter, pragmatic, randomized, cross-over trial (PeLoGAIT). *BMC Pediatrics* **2017**, *17*, 64. [CrossRef]
23. Schoenrath, F.; Markendorf, S.; Brauchlin, A.E.; Seifert, B.; Wilhelm, M.J.; Czerny, M.; Riener, R.; Falk, V.; Schmied, C.M. Robot-Assisted Training Early after Cardiac Surgery. *J. Card. Surg.* **2015**, *30*, 574–580. [CrossRef] [PubMed]
24. Chang, W.H.; Kim, Y.H. Robot-assisted therapy in stroke rehabilitation. *J. Stroke* **2013**, *15*, 174. [CrossRef] [PubMed]
25. Franceschini, M.; Mazzoleni, S.; Goffredo, M.; Pournajaf, S.; Galafate, D.; Criscuolo, S.; Agosti, M.; Posteraro, F. Upper limb robot-assisted rehabilitation versus physical therapy on subacute stroke patients: A follow-up study. *J. Bodyw. Mov. Ther.* **2020**, *1*, 194–208. [CrossRef] [PubMed]
26. Belas dos Santos, M.; Barros de Oliveira, C.; Dos Santos, A.; Garabello Pires, C.; Dylewski, V.; Arida, R.M. A comparative study of conventional physiotherapy versus robot-assisted gait training associated to physiotherapy in individuals with ataxia after stroke. *Behav. Neurol.* **2018**, *2018*, 2892065. [CrossRef] [PubMed]
27. Ferreira, F.M.; Chaves, M.E.; Oliveira, V.C.; Martins, J.S.; Vimieiro, C.; Van Petten, A.M. Effect of Robot-Assisted Therapy on Participation of People with Limited Upper Limb Functioning: A Systematic Review with GRADE Recommendations. *Occup. Ther. Int.* **2021**, *2021*, 6649549. [CrossRef]
28. Villafañe, J.H.; Taveggia, G.; Galeri, S.; Bissolotti, L.; Mullè, C.; Imperio, G.; Valdes, K.; Borboni, A.; Negrini, S. Efficacy of short-term robot-assisted rehabilitation in patients with hand paralysis after stroke: A randomized clinical trial. *Hand* **2018**, *13*, 95–102. [CrossRef]
29. Hátlová, B.; Fleischmann, O.; Chytrý, V. Osobnost a aktivní životní styl seniorů ve věku 65–75 let. *Psychol. A Její Kontexty (Psychol. Its Contexts)* **2017**, *8*, 41–53.
30. Gras, G.; Vitiello, V.; Yang, G.Z. Cooperative control of a compliant manipulator for robotic-assisted physiotherapy. In Proceedings of the 2014IEEE International Conference on Robotics and Automation (ICRA), 31 May–7 June, Hong Kong, China; pp. 339–346.
31. Iosa, M.; Morone, G.; Bragoni, M.; De Angelis, D.; Venturiero, V.; Coiro, P.; Pratesi, L.; Paolucci, S. Driving electromechanically assisted Gait Trainer for people with stroke. *J. Rehabil. Res. Dev.* **2011**, *48*, 135–146. [CrossRef]
32. Rocon, E.; Pons, J.L. *Exoskeletons in Rehabilitation Robotics: Tremor Suppression*; Springer: Berlin/Heidelberg, Germany, 2011; Volume 69.
33. Glowinski, S.; Obst, M.; Majdanik, S.; Potocka-Banaś, B. Dynamic model of a humanoid exoskeleton of a lower limb with hydraulic actuators. *Sensors* **2021**, *21*, 3432. [CrossRef]
34. Flemr, L. *Pohybové Aktivity Ve Vědě a Praxis*; Karolinum Press: Prague, Czech Republic, 2014; ISBN 978-80-246-2621-5.
35. Bayon, C.; Raya, R.; Lara, S.L.; Ramirez, O.; Serrano, J.; Rocon, E. Robotic therapies for children with cerebral palsy: A systematic review. *Transl. Biomed.* **2016**, *7*, 44. [CrossRef]
36. Baňárová, P.; Petríková-Rosiová, I.; Durcová, A. Ako motivovať ľudí k pravidelnému cvičeniu v rámci primárnej prevencie vzniku vertebrogénnych porúch funkčného pôvodu. *Rehabilitácia* **2016**, *53*, 25–34.

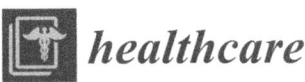 healthcare

Perspective

Information Security in Medical Robotics: A Survey on the Level of Training, Awareness and Use of the Physiotherapist

Lisa Monoscalco [1], Rossella Simeoni [2], Giovanni Maccioni [3] and Daniele Giansanti [3,*]

1. Faculty of Engineering, Tor Vergata University, Via Cracovia, 00133 Rome, Italy; lisamonoscalco@hotmail.com
2. Facoltà di Medicina e Chirurgia, Università Cattolica del Sacro Cuore, Largo Francesco Vito, 1, 00168 Rome, Italy; rossella.simeoni.1955@gmail.com
3. Centre Tisp, Istituto Superiore di Sanità, 00161 Rome, Italy; giovanni.maccioni@iss.it
* Correspondence: Daniele.giansanti@iss.it; Tel.: +39-06-49902701

Abstract: Cybersecurity is becoming an increasingly important aspect to investigate for the adoption and use of care robots, in term of both patients' safety, and the availability, integrity and privacy of their data. This study focuses on opinions about cybersecurity relevance and related skills for physiotherapists involved in rehabilitation and assistance thanks to the aid of robotics. The goal was to investigate the awareness among insiders about some facets of cybersecurity concerning human–robot interactions. We designed an electronic questionnaire and submitted it to a relevant sample of physiotherapists. The questionnaire allowed us to collect data related to: (i) use of robots and its relationship with cybersecurity in the context of physiotherapy; (ii) training in cybersecurity and robotics for the insiders; (iii) insiders' self-assessment on cybersecurity and robotics in some usage scenarios, and (iv) their experiences of cyber-attacks in this area and proposals for improvement. Besides contributing some specific statistics, the study highlights the importance of both acculturation processes in this field and monitoring initiatives based on surveys. The study exposes direct suggestions for continuation of these types of investigations in the context of scientific societies operating in the rehabilitation and assistance robotics. The study also shows the need to stimulate similar initiatives in other sectors of medical robotics (robotic surgery, care and socially assistive robots, rehabilitation systems, training for health and care workers) involving insiders.

Keywords: medical devices; rehabilitation; assistance; robotics; cyber security

Citation: Monoscalco, L.; Simeoni, R.; Maccioni, G.; Giansanti, D. Information Security in Medical Robotics: A Survey on the Level of Training, Awareness and Use of the Physiotherapist. *Healthcare* 2022, 10, 159. https://doi.org/10.3390/healthcare10010159

Academic Editor: Tin-Chih Toly Chen

Received: 3 November 2021
Accepted: 6 January 2022
Published: 14 January 2022

Publisher's Note: MDPI stays neutral with regard to jurisdictional claims in published maps and institutional affiliations.

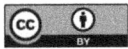

Copyright: © 2022 by the authors. Licensee MDPI, Basel, Switzerland. This article is an open access article distributed under the terms and conditions of the Creative Commons Attribution (CC BY) license (https://creativecommons.org/licenses/by/4.0/).

1. Introduction

Cybersecurity (*Cyb*) in healthcare (*CybH*) includes all the general actions that we can find in the world of industry and consumption (*network security, application security, information security, operational security, disaster recovery and operational continuity, end-user training*), adjusted specifically for the *health domain* [1,2].

CybH addresses the cyber risk in a *cyber-system* in the *health domain*. The *cyber-system* can either be a complex medical device and/or a complex interoperable and heterogeneous system (e.g., a hospital information system, a radiology information system; a dedicated medical network). Important issues emerge for medical devices (MDs).

In the case of a *standalone medical device (SMD)* (not connected to other systems) *CybH* must concentrate on the device itself. Much of the Cyb depends on the correct implementation of the certification processes, considering also the CybH.

If the device *is not standalone, i.e., it is an interconnected Medical Device* (IMD), in addition to a certification process, it is also necessary to consider the *Cyb* vulnerability of the IT environment (e.g., hospital information system, the network of the rehabilitation centre, the home WI-FI).

Nowadays, it is rare to find SMDs. Most MDs are IMDs. Examples are the *artificial pancreas* and the *pacemaker*. They need a communication link to an IT environment, both for the monitoring and/or updating functions [3–6].

Medical robots used in rehabilitation and assistance [7,8] are examples of IMDs: they need a communication link to exchange and record data, for updating and and/or other functions.

1.1. Regulatory and Legislative Issues in Medical Robotics

Safety and security concepts are at the base of the *Cyb* of rehabilitation and assistance robots.

In general, when we talk about safety we must distinguish well between safety and security [9]. The term "safety" concerns protections and countermeasures against actions, conditions or circumstances that could harm (physically and/or psychologically) living beings, and particularly humans (see for example the IETF Internet Security Glossary [10]). The term "security" is sometimes used as a broader term encompassing "safety"; however, it is more often used in relation to assets more diverse than living beings, such as data, networks, computers, and money. In the context of cyber-physical systems, the term usually refers to data, hardware, or computing processes. The typical case of using the robot is as an IMD in the hospital (or similar facility) or at home. Therefore, regarding IMD robot safety and security, the medical device itself, the environments of use (for example, the hospital or the home), and the organization and working regulations must be taken into consideration.

The problem is very broad and includes: (a) the safety of the patient and the worker (e.g., the physiotherapist); (b) the regulations for the medical devices; (c) the regulations for the safe use of networks; and (d) other interrelated regulations, such as product safety in general or radio directives. Both work safety and patient safety in Europe present a very complex regulation framework. In any case, the employer/hospital manager is always responsible for both safety and security (from delinquent actions) and this applies also to *cyber-systems*.

The European Union has recently recalled the entire existing regulation framework [11] through a Communication from the Commission to the European Parliament, the Council, the European Economic and Social Committee and the Committee of Regions. This Communication regards the practical implementation of the provisions of the Health and Safety at Work Directives [11]. In [12], an examination of the European regulations on patient safety and, more generally, hospital safety is reported.

Fosch-Villaronga and Mahler provided in their recent study [13] a very fine analysis in this direction, for the European framework, identifying problems and criticisms with regard to points (b) to (d) above. *As a first step,* they considered the relationship between robots in the *health domain* and the European general product safety regulations (*Directive 2001/95/EC of the European Parliament and of the Council of 3 December 2001 on general product safety 2001, and Directive 85/374/EEC on liability for defective products*) [14].

They highlighted that the applicability of product liability laws is not straightforward for the robots, comprising cyber-physical systems.

As a second step, they analyzed the impact of the medical device regulation (MDR) (Regulation (EU) 2017/745) [15] on the robots.

Finally, they focused on the three legal frameworks partially regulating robot *Cyb* (NIS Directive, GDPR, Cybersecurity ACT) [16–18] both as MD and IMD interconnected to a network. The scholars reported that also other regulations impacted on *Cyb*. They gave the example of the EU Radio Equipment Directive [19].

The authors highlighted [13] the novelty of the MDR. They also highlighted the *shadows*. The *first shadow* is that MDR focuses heavily on manufacturers and little on recipients/users. The *second shadow* is that compliance with cybersecurity requirements is challenging, due to the potential overlap of different certification schemes (with varying geographical or product scope) and to the evolution of regulations external to the MDR [14].

The *third shadow* is that the specific *Cyb* certifications are voluntary, as in the case of the *cybersecurity ACT* [18]. We found another important *shadow*. The intended use and certification as MD do not always seem aligned (for example when MDs used in rehabilitation are not certified for this) [20]. *Cyber-attacks can have serious physical and/or psychological impacts* [12], as described by means of a model in [13].

1.2. The Medical Robots Used in Rehabilitation and Assistance and Cybersecurity

An important sector for medical robots is that of rehabilitation and assistance. Robotics in rehabilitation [7,21–31] essentially concerns three sectors:

- Balance (BA)
- The lower limbs (LOLI)
- The upper limbs (UPLI)

These sectors use *exoskeleton* or *end-effector technology*. The exoskeletal robot completely covers the limb, following and replicating the human anthropometry. The mechanics guide each segment involved in the rehabilitation practice. Therefore, an exoskeleton is a "mechatronic" apparatus. It is worn and performs the same kinematic/dynamic activity practiced by the patient. In a robotic end-effector device, the input for carrying out the rehabilitation exercise comes directly from the distal part of the limb. It allows the natural kinematic activation of the movement, without unnatural constraints.

Assistance robotics uses "social robots" (SRs) [8,32]. Use of these devices has recently increased, to overcome the problem of social distancing in the Covid-19 pandemic.

Today, SRs are designed to:

- Interact with people, even by touching them, since the physical contact helps to establish a better emotional relationship.
- Assist people with many daily activities (as a reminder or as a kind of butler).
- Assist people in medical activities, such as drug administration and patient monitoring.
- Support physicians in physical rehabilitation, such as *Pepper*, which supports physiotherapists during sessions [33–36], or support patients in their movements or displacements (e.g., *Robear* [37,38] transports patients).
- Support people with complex communication needs.
- Support families or therapists as cultural mediators.

The SRs are a totally new challenge for *CybH*. There are important aspects related to *Cyb* that require consideration in these devices, since their programming has important implications for the robot's moral behaviour, resulting in the interdisciplinary field of machine ethics [39–45]—that is, how to program robots with ethical rules [40].

This sector involves "adding an ethical dimension to the machine" [45], and it has become of utmost importance because of wonderful technological developments in the field of the CRs and, more generally, artificial intelligence [41–45]. Gordon [39] highlighted that making ethics "computable" depends in part on how the designers understand ethics and attempt to implement that understanding in programs, but also on their expertise in the field of human–robot interaction. He found that researchers and programmers have neither a good enough understanding nor sufficient ethical expertise to build moral machines that would be comparable to human beings with respect to ethical reasoning and decision-making. Figure 1 shows the modelling of the physical and psychological impact [13], developed by us for the rehabilitation and assistance robotics. Note that psychological harm can also occur as an indirect consequence of physical damage or harm caused by rehabilitation robots. It is therefore clear that there is a strong need for studies to help develop consensus in this area. It is important to stimulate the stakeholders to face these problems. It is also important to sensitize scholars to invest energies in research initiatives.

1.3. Motivation and Purpose of the Study

It is vital to plan an acculturalization process on *Cyb*. This process must concern all the actors involved, from the builders up to the users and the caregivers, in the different environments (from home up to the hospital).

Training in this area must also become an important issue. Stakeholders will have to start specific monitoring initiatives, through targeted surveys, for example, to verify the state of diffusion of the *Cyb* culture in robotics, and assess the consensus and opinion in this area. This is an important and preliminary step in the launch of agreements and consensus initiatives for these devices, also considering that *Cyb* certification of CRs is voluntary. At present, there are no active initiatives of this type. A search on Pubmed with the key *"cyber security" [Title/Abstract] AND "robotics" [Title/Abstract] AND "questionnaire" [Title/Abstract]* (also trying with synonyms) did not show results.

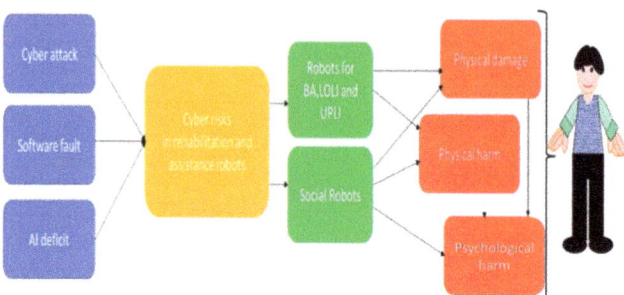

Figure 1. Model of the impact of the cyber-attacks in the investigated field.

In other sectors of the *health domain*, where technology is rapidly developing, ad hoc questionnaires have been developed with the aim of investigating the consensus between the actors. For example, in digital radiology, various studies have focused on different actors and conducted research through questionnaires on a very important issue relating to *information technology in cyber-systems*, that of *artificial intelligence*. Selected papers [46–56] highlight studies focused on some of the actors concerned: radiologists and radiographers [49–54], primary care providers [51], students [55], and patients [46–48], that is, both on service providers and users, and on the subjects in training. The importance of training and the usefulness of free questionnaires emerged from these studies. Surveys were used both to collect interviews and structured data from focus groups/consensus initiatives. In all cases identified, original questionnaires based on choice questions Likert scales, graded questions (in a psychometric scale) and open-ended questions were used. With very few exceptions [48], scholars preferred to use personal and original rather than validated/standardized questionnaires to investigate the topic.

For this reason, we consider a similar approach as regards robot technology (also rapidly evolving) to be useful on another topic connected to *information technology in cyber-systems*, that of *Cyb*, where, similarly, training plays a leading role. For this reason, we believe it is equally useful to propose it to the professionals involved in this area.

Many professionals in the *health domain* have to do with the robots in rehabilitation and assistance (from the bioengineer up to the physiotherapist). The physiotherapists are key professionals in this field. It is therefore important to investigate the relationship between the physiotherapist and *CybH*.

This is useful to provide *medical knowledge* and stimulate stakeholders to recommend initiatives.

We have therefore set ourselves the goal to focus on the physiotherapist and: (1) to investigate the consensus, familiarity, and opinion on *Cyb* in this field, based both on the training and experience in the *workplace*; (2) to apply an electronic questionnaire designed for the investigation.

2. Materials and Methods

In line with the aim of the study, we decided to develop an electronic questionnaire to investigate the acceptance and the consensus of the physiotherapists. We used Microsoft Forms (Microsoft Corporation, Albuquerque, Nuovo Mexico (NM), USA), available in the Microsoft 365 App Business Premium suite in the *workplace*. It is the software product recommended by the company's Data Protection Office (DPO). It is included in the informatic domain and complies to the regulations on data privacy and security. We adhered to the *SURGE Checklist* [57] for the development and administration of the questionnaire. The questionnaire used different type of questions: *open questions, choice questions, multiple choice questions, Likert scales, graded questions*. A six-level psychometric scale was used both in the graded questions and in the Likerts. Therefore, it was possible to assign a minimum score of one and a maximum score of six. The theoretical mean value (TMV) was equal to 3.5. We used the TMV for comparison in the analysis: an average value below the TMV shows a more negative than positive response, whereas an average value above TMV indicates a more positive than negative response.

For the check of data normality, we used the Kolmogorov–Smirnov test, which is preferable for sample sizes like ours. The software SPSS V. 25.0 (IBM SPSS software, Armonk, NY, USA) was used in the study. The Cohen's d effect size estimated with 0.499 the effect size. A sample with $n > 60$ was estimated to be suitable for the study. We submitted the survey from 1 June 2021 until 20 October 2021.

We have submitted the questionnaire to the physiotherapists using social networks, web sources, messengers, and lists/webs from professional associations.

Figure 2 reports the diagram of the inclusion process. Table 1 shows the demographic characteristics.

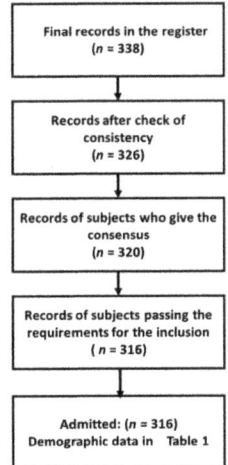

Figure 2. Diagram describing the inclusion process.

Table 1. Characteristics of the participants.

Submission	Participants	Males/Females	Min Age/Max Age	Mean Age
Physiotherapists	316	162/154	23/58	38.47

The methodology, based on an electronic survey, focused on the physiotherapist. It investigated, through the tools available in the survey, the different aspects of *Cyb*.

The electronic survey is arranged into five sections (see Table 2).

Table 2. Sections of the questionnaire.

Section	Title
Section 1	Demographic data
Section 2	Robotics and cybersecurity in the workplace
Section 3	Training in cybersecurity and robotics
Section 4	Self-assessment on cybersecurity and robotics
Section 5	Proposals and collection of personal cases of cyber-risk

Section 1 is designed for collecting the demographic data (reported in Table 1). *Section 2* investigates if there is an interaction with the robots in the workplace and whether this interaction also concerns *Cyb*. *Section 3* investigates the specific training on *Cyb* and on the connected disciplines. *Section 4* proposes *self-assessment* questions regarding *Cyb* while interacting with the robots. *Section 5* collects both proposals and the cyber-risk experiences in one's work environment useful both for the reader and the stakeholder.

3. Results

The results are reported in the four sections below. For each section, the type of questions, the questions asked, and the statistics are reported.

3.1. Output from Section 2 "Robotics and Cybersecurity in the Workplace"

As a first aspect, we investigated the use of rehabilitation robotics and the involvement (role) of physiotherapists in its use, either as active users or just observers. A *multiple-choice* question was proposed (relating to three different robots used in rehabilitation).

Figure 3 shows that only 102 (32.27%) respondents use rehabilitation robotics in the *workplace*. In detail, 73 (23.10%) use robotics in upper limb rehabilitation. A smaller number use robotics in the other two sectors of balance (54, 17.08%) and lower limb rehabilitation (51, 16.14%).

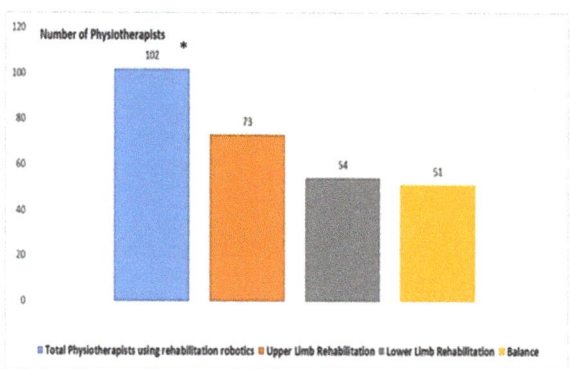

Figure 3. Use of rehabilitation robotics in the *workplace* (* 102 is different from the sum of the three choices, because it is a multiple-choice question).

A second question with two choices (Yes/No) also investigated involvement in *Cyb* activity.

Figure 4 highlights that all the interviewed people reported the role of technology user. Only 29 (9.18%) claimed to have been involved in the *CybH*, resulting in a significantly low number (p-Value < 0.01, χ^2 test).

It is well known that the use of SR is still very limited. However, we wanted to investigate any involvement, which could also concern research projects. Three questions were proposed. A question with two choices (Yes/No) investigated the SR presence in the *workplace*. A question with two choices (*only observer/user*) investigated the role in the interaction. A question on their role in *Cyb* was also proposed to those who had responded "user". Figure 5 highlights that only 5 respondents stated that they were dealing with SRs. Three (0.95%) declared that they were observers, two (0.63%) were users, and only one (0.32%) faced *CybH* issues. These frequencies also had a high statistical significance (p-value < 0.01, χ^2 test).

3.2. Output from Section 3 "Training in Cybersecurity and Robotics"

Table 3 reports *the perceived level of training on SRs, robots for BA, robots for LOLI, robots for UPLI*. Four graded questions with 6 levels of score (1 = min; 6 = max) were used.

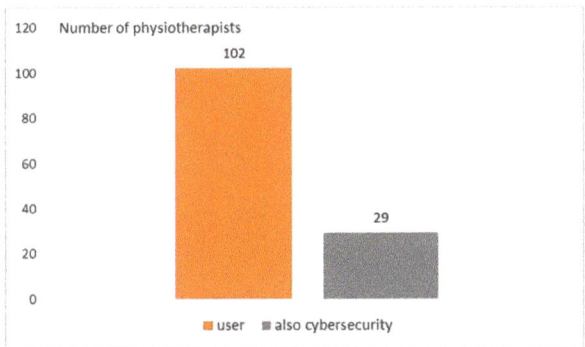

Figure 4. Role of the use of rehabilitation robotics by physiotherapists.

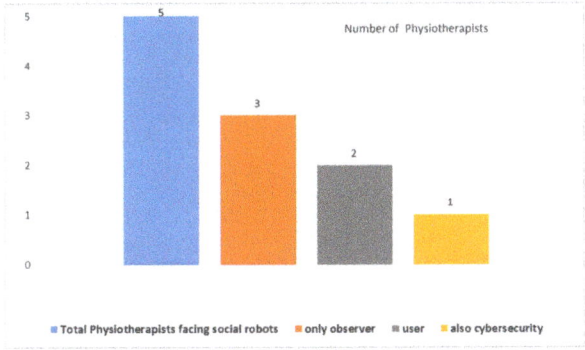

Figure 5. Physiotherapists' interaction with social robots.

Table 3. Perceived degree of training on SRs, robots for BA, robots for LOLI, robots for UPLI.

Question	Mean	CI 95%
Upper limb rehabilitation	4.55	±0.38
Lower limb rehabilitation	4.43	±0.37
Balance	4.42	±0.38
Social robot	3.63	±0.38

The most popular response was *Robots* for UPLI. The least popular answer was *Social Robots*. All the answers received a score above the TMV.

Table 4 reports the *Perceived training on informatics, mHealth, eHealth, cybersecurity*. Four graded questions with 6 levels of score (1 = min; 6 = max) were used.

Table 4. Perceived degree of training on informatics, mHealth, eHealth, cybersecurity.

Question	Mean	CI 95%
Informatics	4.57	±0.38
Electronic health	4.41	±0.37
Mobile health	4.45	±0.37
Cybersecurity	2.49	±0.36

The most popular response was *informatics*. The least popular answer was *Cyb*. All the answers obtained a score above the TMV except for *Cyb*.

Table 5 reports the perceived training on *Cyb* with reference to the different cyber-attacks. A Likert scale was used with the modules associated to each cyber-attack. Each module had 6 levels (1 = min; 6 = max). Results show low scores, all below the TMV, except for *malware, phishing, and password crackers* (just above the threshold).

Table 5. Assessed knowledge on cybersecurity.

Question	Mean	CI 95%
Malware (virus, Trojan, ransomware, scareware...)	3.57	±0.36
Man in the middle	2.41	±0.37
Denial of service (DoS)	2.45	±0.38
Distributed denial of service (DDoS)	2.49	±0.35
Spoofing	2.46	±0.38
Sniffing	3.13	±0.37
Phishing	3.60	±0.38
Data breach	2.46	±0.37
Back door	2.46	±0.33
Password cracker	3.56	±0.32

We asked also to indicate (*based on the training*) *the sector mostly affected by the problem of Cyb*. A Likert scale was used with the modules associated to each robot. Each module had 6 levels (1 = min; 6 = max). Table 6 reports the responses related to the specific Likert scale. The most popular response was the SR. The least popular answer was the BA. All the answers received a score above the TMV.

Table 6. Perception on the influence of Cyb in Robotics.

Question	Mean	CI 95%
SR	4.58	±0.38
BA	3.87	±0.37
UPLI	4.21	±0.37
LOLI	4.22	±0.36

We completed this section asking specific further questions on the regulatory issues and on the awareness of the role with *Cyb*. Two graded questions with 6 levels of score (1 = min; 6 = max) were used for investigating the training on regulatory issues. The first question investigated the training on the regulatory issues on *Cyb*. The second question investigated the training on the regulatory issues on *Cyb*, specifically referring to robotics.

Figure 6 highlights a very low level of training on regulatory issues both as a whole (average value = 2.89; confidence interval (CI) 95%: ±0.35) and related to robotics (average value = 2.88; CI 95%: ±0.35). Two graded questions with 6 levels of score (1 = min; 6 = max) were used for investigating awareness on their role with *Cyb*. The first question investigated the awareness of the role with *Cyb*. The second question investigated awareness of the role with *Cyb* and robotics. Figure 7 highlights a level of awareness well above the TMV (with reference to the role of the physiotherapist in *Cyb* as a whole (average value = 4.31; CI 95%: ±0.38) and while interacting with robotics (average value = 3.98; CI 95%: ±0.37).

3.3. Output from Section 4 "Self-Assessment on Cybersecurity and Robotics"

This section considers the self-assessment scenarios of familiarity with *Cyb*. *A first investigation* involved a mapping of cyber-attacks in relation to the four robots (Table 7). Each one of the cyber-attacks was proposed with *multiple choices* (LOLI, UPLI, BA, SR). The interviewees could indicate the applicability or non-applicability of cyber-attacks with the robots. Table 6 highlights how *malware, phishing and password crackers* were the most indicated. However, a statistical frequency analysis did not show significance ($\chi 2$test, *p*-Value = 0.221).

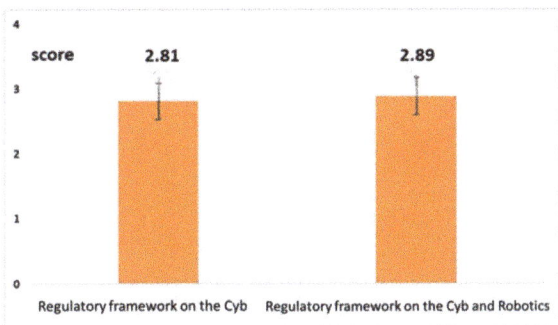

Figure 6. Level of training on the regulatory framework (also referred to robotics).

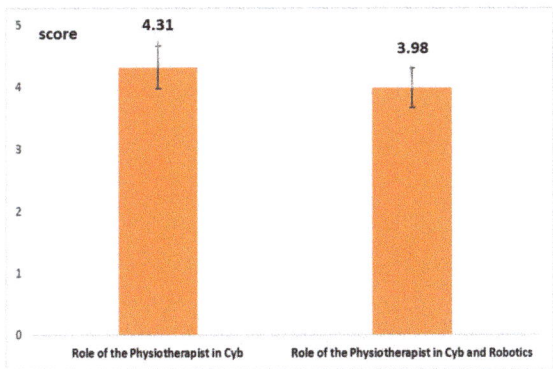

Figure 7. Level of awareness on the role of the physiotherapist on Cyb.

Table 7. Results relating to the graded questions with the details of the assessment.

Question	BA	LOLI	UPLI	SR
Malware (virus, Trojan, ransomware, scareware...)	310	309	311	308
Man in the middle	251	247	259	253
Denial of service (DoS)	252	261	249	248
Distributed denial of service (DDoS)	249	252	253	250
Spoofing	247	250	252	249
Sniffing	278	281	293	300
Phishing	309	310	310	312
Data breach	279	268	269	288
Back door	269	257	258	267
Password cracker	309	309	3011	312

A second investigation (Table 8) concerned the model proposed in Figure 1. The functional problems (*physical damage, physical harm, physiological harm*) were proposed with *multiple choices* (LOLI, UPLI, BA, SR). The SRs showed the lowest scores for *physical harm*, with statistical significance (χ^2test, *p*-Value = 0.048) and physical damage with statistical significance (χ^2test, *p*-Value = 0.049). However, the SRs showed the highest score for *psychological harm*, with a high statistical significance (χ^2test, *p*-Value = 0.008).

As *a third investigation* we proposed a specific risk self-assessment (Tables 9–12). A Likert scale was proposed for each one of the robots (UPLI, LOLI, BA, SR). The modules in the Likert were identical. Each module had 6 levels of score (1 = min; 6 = max). The scores almost overlapped and were above the TMV for UPLI, LOLI, BA. For these robots the scenario "On the possible effect on the patient/practitioner's health and safety" obtained the highest score. All the values were below the threshold for the SRs, except for the score associated with the scenario "On the possible effect on the patient/practitioner's health and safety".

Table 8. Results relating to the graded questions with the details of the assessment.

	BA	LOLI	UPLI	SR
Physical damage	308	309	307	212
Physical harm	307	306	305	213
Psychological harm	13	14	18	309

Table 9. Level of awareness in cyber-risk scenarios for UPLI.

Level of Awareness	Mean	CI 95%
During software update process	3.89	±0.37
During upload process	3.92	±0.38
General vulnerability	3.63	±0.37
On the possible effect on the patient/practitioner's health and safety	4.39	±0.33

Table 10. Level of awareness in cyber-risk scenarios for LOLI.

Level of Awareness	Mean	CI 95%
During software update process	3.88	±0.37
During upload process	3.99	±0.38
General vulnerability	3.64	±0.37
On the possible effect on the patient/practitioner's health and safety	4.39	±0.33

Table 11. Level of awareness in cyber-risk scenarios for BA.

Level of Awareness	Mean	CI 95%
During software update process	3.89	±0.37
During upload process	3.95	±0.38
General vulnerability	3.57	±0.37
On the possible effect on the patient/practitioner's health and safety	4.41	±0.33

Table 12. Level of awareness in cyber-risk scenarios for SR.

Level of Awareness	Mean	CI 95%
During software update process	3.47	±0.39
During upload process	3.44	±0.43
General vulnerability	3.45	±0.41
On the possible effect on the patient/practitioner's health and safety	4.28	±0.41

3.4. Output from Section 5 "Proposals and Collection of Personal Experiences of Cyber-Risk"

As *a final investigation* we have invited respondents to: (a) freely express opinions and suggestions on cyber-risks and actions to consider shortly; (b) cite personal experiences related to *Cyb* problems. Open-ended questions were used in this section.

3.4.1. Proposals

We grouped and categorized similar questions. Table 13 reports the suggestions for the most probable cyber risks to face. The most worrying concern was the *physical damage* caused by an incorrect imposition of motion. Table 14 reports the suggestions related to the actions to consider. The most suggested action was related to the periodic monitoring activities managed by the scientific societies.

Table 13. Suggestions on the cyber risk to face.

Priority	Suggestion	Number of Suggestions
1	Risk of physical damage for incorrect imposition of kinematic/dynamic therapy	89
2	Risk of incorrect recording of the trials	72
3	Risk of out-of-control behavior of the SR	16

Table 14. Suggestions on the actions to consider.

Priority	Suggestion	Number of Suggestions
1	Launch periodic monitoring actions led by scientific societies.	83
2	Create heterogeneous national working groups to address cybersecurity in the 4 sectors of robotics	46
3	Launch training initiatives on the various issues of cybersecurity applied to the various sectors of robotics.	26

3.4.2. Collection of Personal Experiences of Cyber-Risk

We also invited the physiotherapists to describe an experience in this field. There was an open space of about a half page of space for this. Both the participants with a direct experience on robotics and the participants with only a training experience contributed with enthusiasm. 302 (95.57%) physiotherapists described an experience of a problem with *Cyb* in the workplace. 55 participants reported *Cyb* problems with robotics in the workplace. We should consider that in *Section 2* (see Section 3.1) it emerged that 102 physiotherapists work with rehabilitative robotics and 2 deal with SRs as users. This means that 52.3% of them were involved in a *Cyb* problem.

The problems have been analyzed and categorized. The problems that occurred more than one time are shown in Figure 8. Figure 8 highlights how the two most frequent reported and described attacks were the *denial of service* (7 times), which involved a network with LOLI, UPLI, BA, and ransomware attacks on the data of a LOLI platform (5 times).

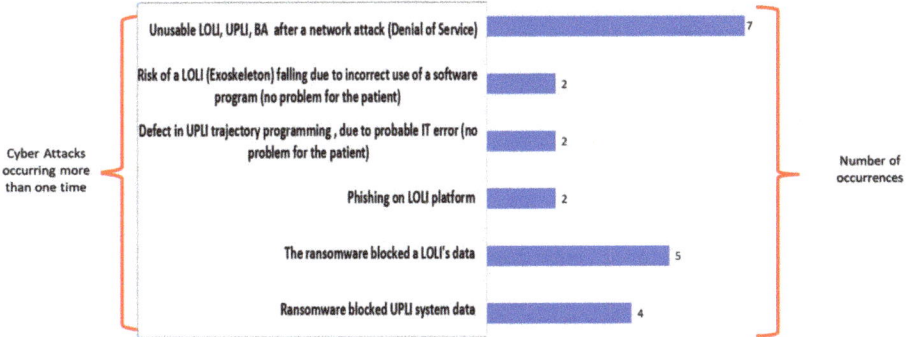

Figure 8. Experiences with cyber-attacks which occurred more than one time after categorization.

4. Discussion

Mechatronic devices have grown in importance in recent years [7,24]. Among these devices we certainly find the robots for rehabilitation and assistance [8,21–32]. The increased use of these technologies raises important issues on *Cyb*. It is important to investigate the perceptions of the insiders, also in robotics, as for other disruptive technologies [58].

We started with the physiotherapist, who is facing a transformation towards digitalization in the pandemic era, as has been highlighted by A. Lee in [59].

In this study we have proposed a useful electronic questionnaire. It included: *open-ended questions, choice questions, multiple choice questions, Likert scales, and graded questions*. It permitted collection of important data on: *(a) the use of robotics and direct involvement in the CybH; (b) training in robotics, cybersecurity, and other disciplines; (c) self-perception of cybersecurity and robotics; (d) opinions, suggestions, and experiences.*

When we place our investigation in the international context, we must consider the following. *Cyb* has vast implications in the *health domain* and it is evident that it has been the subject of many targeted studies [60]. However, the number of the studies focusing also on robotics is extremely low [61]. The research [60] in Pubmed (the most important database of the *health domain*) shows that, to date, no one has yet addressed specific issues of *Cyb* in robotics, submitting questionnaires to medical professionals.

The questionnaire, dedicated to physiotherapists and with reference to *CybH* in robotics, has the advantage of allowing the monitoring of roles and interactions in the workplace, monitoring of training received, a self-assessment of risks, and a virtual focus group.

The study has some limitations. *A first limitation* is that the questionnaire is both dedicated to one field of the medical robotics (the rehabilitation and assistance robotics) and calibrated on a professional group. Many professional groups play an important role in rehabilitation and assistance robotics. Specialized questionnaires for these professional groups should be developed in the future.

Another second limitation is the limitlessness of the theme. It is impossible to address all the implications in a single study.

In particular, the ethical implications of robotics are very important. These implications will have a strong impact on *Cyb* and require a very robust and multidisciplinary approach involving all the actors.

There are two important macro-sectors of ethics with an impact on *Cyb*. The first macro-sector is the ethics in a responsible research and innovation [62]. Stahl and Coeckelbergh highlighted, for the first macro-sector, the important implications of *Cyb* [63–70] in the replacement of the human in work, as regards the responsibility for and in the management of information. The second macro-sector is the ethics problem encountered while building moral robots [39]. This focuses on the interdisciplinary field of machine ethics.

The *third limitation* is that the questionnaire (which allows important feedback for the stakeholders) represents only a first scientific step. The subsequent steps that this study aims to stimulate are the integration of this questionnaire together with other solutions during the application of agreement initiatives. The Consensus Conferences [71–73], for example, could be an important agreement initiative and could certainly benefit (in the context of the activities of the working groups [74–76]) from the use of electronic questionnaires that provide for structured feedback and virtual focus groups.

Our questionnaire has the above-listed limits. However, it *has the merit* of having initiated this approach, in a delicate issue (*medical robotics*), and of being a stimulus for the *scientific societies involved*. It is in line with other similar initiatives in the *health domain*. International scientific meetings, promoted *by scientific societies* [77], now include sections dedicated to the problems of *Cyb* in the HCI. In a study [78], just presented in [77], the importance of using dedicated surveys is stressed, to improve understanding of behaviors at risk, as regards *Cyb*, when using HCI in the *health domain*. Our study is in this direction. Likewise, it addresses the *Cyb* problems in a new field of the HCI, the human robot interaction (a complex HCI with mechatronics) [79], through a wide-ranging investigation, using a questionnaire and involving concerned actors..

5. Conclusions

Rehabilitation and assistance robots represent an opportunity for the health domain [7,8]. The use of these robots has important implications. They can be used with fragile patients or people with disabilities, in rehabilitation and assistance processes. They can be used in psychological and cognitive rehabilitation processes for children and other subjects with communication disabilities, as in the case of SRs. Therefore, their use can have important physical and psychological implications. Furthermore, the software in these devices interact with sensible data. Cybersecurity has therefore become an important issue to face, starting from the insiders. We have proposed an investigation based on a questionnaire submitted to physiotherapists. The investigation showed the following highlights:

- The questionnaire, dedicated to physiotherapists and with reference to *CybH* in robotics, has the advantage of allowing a monitoring of roles and interactions in the workplace, a monitoring of training received, a self-assessment of risks, and a virtual focus group.
- The questions enabled us to collect important data on: (a) the use of robotics and the direct involvement in *CybH*; (b) training in robotics, cybersecurity, and other disciplines; (c) the self-perception of *Cyb* and robotics; (d) opinions, suggestions, and experiences.
- The data concerned both subjects with only training experiences and subjects with direct work experience.
- At the time of the survey, 102 (32.27%) respondents used rehabilitation robotics in the workplace. All have highlighted their role as user, but only 29 (9.18%) had a direct involvement with *Cyb*. Only 5 respondents stated that they were dealing with SRs. Of these, 3 (0.95%) were observers and 2 (0.63%) were users, while only one (0.32%) had a direct involvement in *Cyb*.
- An acceptable training regarding robotics and other related training modules. An unacceptable training when dealing, in detail, with *Cyb* issues. A training that highlighted gaps for the regulation issues on *Cyb* (also referred to robotics). An awareness, during the training, on the involvement of the physiotherapist in *Cyb* (also related to robotics).
- The possibility for physiotherapists to self-assess themselves in some *Cyb* scenarios proposed in respect of robots.
- Opinions on emerging risks and wishes in this field (as, for example, to continue the use of the questionnaire and to create specific working groups). Both the participants with a direct experience of robotics and participants with only a training experience narrated experiences in this field with enthusiasm: 302 (95.57%) described their experiences with robotics, categorized after data mining, showing that 55 reported *Cyb* problems with robotics in the *workplace*. This, very importantly, highlighted that 52.3% of the physiotherapists engaged with robotics in the workplace reported a *Cyb* problem. The most frequent incidents were *denial of service* (7), which involved a network with LOLI, UPLI, BA, and ransomware attacks on the data of a LOLI platform (5).

6. Future Work

The needs for future work that emerge from this study concern both continuation in the field of rehabilitation and assistance robotics and the activation of similar initiatives in other sectors of robotics.

6.1. Future Initiatives in the Field of Rehabilitation and Assistance Robotics

Future developments of this study are foreseen to include:

- An improvement of the electronic questionnaire, with a standardization of the same, interacting with the scientific societies;
- Using it for specific periodic monitoring and investigations;

- Stimulating the stakeholders for the creation of multidisciplinary workgroups to address *Cyb* (ranging from engineering to machine ethics, legal and policy issues);
- Expansion to other professional groups.

6.2. Suggestions for Future Developments in Other Sectors of Medical Robotics

The Policy Department for Economic, Scientific and Quality of Life Policies, of the European Parliament, identified the most interesting applications for the medical robots [79]: *Robotic surgery, care and socially assistive robots, rehabilitation systems, training for health and care workers*. The sector is wide, complex and with numerous implications for CybH. What emerged in this study may be a stimulus for those engaged in other areas of medical robotics to initiate similar studies focused on *Cyb*.

Author Contributions: Conceptualization, D.G. and L.M.; methodology, D.G.; software, D.G.; validation, D.G., R.S. and G.M.; formal analysis, D.G.; investigation, L.M., R.S., G.M., D.G.; resources, L.M., R.S., G.M., D.G.; data curation, L.M., R.S., G.M., D.G.; writing—original draft preparation, D.G.; writing—review and editing, L.M., R.S., G.M., D.G.; visualization, L.M., R.S., G.M., D.G.; supervision, L.M., R.S., G.M., D.G.; project administration, L.M., R.S., G.M., D.G. All authors have read and agreed to the published version of the manuscript.

Funding: This research received no external funding.

Institutional Review Board Statement: Not applicable.

Informed Consent Statement: Not applicable.

Data Availability Statement: Not applicable.

Conflicts of Interest: The authors declare no conflict of interest.

References

1. Giansanti, D. Cybersecurity and the Digital-Health: The Challenge of This Millennium. *Healthcare* **2021**, *9*, 62. [CrossRef] [PubMed]
2. Giansanti, D.; Monoscalco, L. The cyber-risk in cardiology: Towards an investigation on the self-perception among the cardiologists. *Mhealth* **2021**, *7*, 28. [CrossRef] [PubMed]
3. Baranchuk, A.; Alexander, B.; Campbell, D.; Haseeb, S.; Redfearn, D.; Simpson, C.; Glover, B. Pacemaker Cybersecurity. *Circulation* **2018**, *138*, 1272–1273. [CrossRef] [PubMed]
4. Kramer, D.B.; Fu, K. Cybersecurity concerns and medical devices: Lessons from a pacemaker advisory. *JAMA* **2017**, *318*, 2077–2078. [CrossRef]
5. O'Keeffe, D.T.; Maraka, S.; Basu, A.; Keith-Hynes, P.; Kudva, Y.C. Cybersecurity in artificial pancreas experiments. *Diabetes Technol. Ther.* **2015**, *17*, 664–666. [CrossRef]
6. Coronado, A.J.; Wong, T.L. Healthcare cybersecurity risk management: Keys to an effective plan. *Biomed. Instrum. Technol.* **2014**, *48* (Suppl. S1), 26–30. [CrossRef]
7. Giansanti, D. The Rehabilitation and the Robotics: Are They Going Together Well? *Health* **2020**, *9*, 26. [CrossRef]
8. Wairagkar, M.; De Lima, M.R.; Harrison, M.; Batey, P.; Daniels, S.; Barnaghi, P.; Sharp, D.J.; Vaidyanathan, R. Conversational artificial intelligence and affective social robot for monitoring health and well-being of people with dementia. *Alzheimer's Dement.* **2021**, *17*, e053276. [CrossRef]
9. Available online: http://www.differencebetween.net/language/words-language/difference-between-safety-and-security/ (accessed on 2 November 2021).
10. Available online: https://www.rfc-editor.org/info/rfc4949 (accessed on 2 November 2021).
11. Communication from the Commission to the European Parliament, the Council, the European Economic and Social Committee and the Committee of Regions on the Practical Implementation of the Provisions of the Health and Safety at Work Directives 89/391 (Framework), 89/654 (Workplaces), 89/655 (Work Equipment), 89/656 (Personal Protective Equipment), 90/269 (Manual Handling of Loads) and 90/270 (Display Screen Equipment). Available online: https://eur-lex.europa.eu/legal-content/EN/ALL/?uri=CELEX%3A52004DC0062 (accessed on 2 November 2021).
12. Pilarska, A.; Zimmermann, A.; Piątkowska, K.; Jabłoński, T. Patient Safety Culture in EU Legislation. *Healthcare* **2020**, *8*, 410. [CrossRef]
13. Fosch-Villaronga, E.; Mahler, T. Safety and robots: Strengthening the link between cybersecurity and safety in the context of care robots. *Comput. Law Secur. Rev.* **2021**, *41*, 105528. [CrossRef]
14. Directive 2001/95/EC of the European Parliament and of the Council of 3 December 2001 on General Product Safety. 2001. Available online: https://eur-lex.europa.eu/legal-content/EN/TXT/?uri=celex%3A32001L0095 (accessed on 2 November 2021).

15. Regulation (EU) 2017/745 of the European Parliament and of the Council of 5 April 2017 on Medical Devices, Amending Directive 2001/83/EC, Regulation (EC) No 178/2002 and Regulation (EC) No 1223/2009 and Repealing Council Directives 90/385/EEC and 93/42/EEC.2017. Available online: https://eur-lex.europa.eu/legal-content/EN/TXT/PDF/?uri=CELEX:32017R0745 (accessed on 2 November 2021).
16. Available online: https://www.itgovernance.eu/fi-fi/nis-directive-fi (accessed on 2 November 2021).
17. Available online: https://gdpr.eu/ (accessed on 2 November 2021).
18. Available online: https://digital-strategy.ec.europa.eu/en/policies/cybersecurity-act (accessed on 2 November 2021).
19. European Commission. Impact Assessment on Increased Protection of Internet-Connected Radio Equipment and Wearable Radio Wquipment. 2020. Available online: https://ec.europa.eu/docsroom/documents/40763/attachments/2/translations/en/renditions/native (accessed on 2 November 2021).
20. Gandolfi, M.; Valè, N.; Posteraro, F.; Morone, G.; Dell'Orco, A.; Botticelli, A.; Dimitrova, E.; Gervasoni, E.; Goffredo, M.; Zenzeri, J.; et al. State of the art and challenges for the classification of studies on electromechanical and robotic devices in neurorehabilitation: A scoping review. *Eur. J. Phys. Rehabil. Med.* **2021**, *57*, 831–840. [CrossRef]
21. Bach-y-Rita, P. Late postacute neurologic rehabilitation: Neuroscience, engineering, and clinical programs. *Arch. Phys. Med. Rehabil.* **2003**, *84*, 1100–1108. [CrossRef]
22. Hidler, J.; Nichols, D.; Pelliccio, M.; Brady, K. Advances in the understanding and treatment of stroke impairment using robotic devices. *Top. Stroke Rehabil.* **2005**, *12*, 22–35. [CrossRef]
23. Volpe, B.T.; Huerta, P.T.; Zipse, J.L.; Rykman, A.; Edwards, D.; Dipietro, L.; Hogan, N.; Krebs, H.I. Robotic devices as therapeutic and diagnostic tools for stroke recovery. *Arch. Neurol.* **2009**, *66*, 1086–1090. [CrossRef]
24. Giansanti, D. *Automatized Rehabilitation of Walking and Posture: Proposals, Problems and Integration into e-Health, Rapporti ISTISAN 18/10*; Istituto Superiore di Sanità: Roma, Italy, 2019; pp. 1–50.
25. Sawicki, G.S.; Beck, O.N.; Kang, I.; Young, A.J. The exoskeleton expansion: Improving walking and running economy. *J. Neuroeng. Rehabil.* **2020**, *17*, 25. [CrossRef]
26. Mehrholz, J.; Pollock, A.; Pohl, M.; Kugler, J.; Elsner, B. Systematic review with network meta-analysis of randomized controlled trials of robotic-assisted arm training for improving activities of daily living and upper limb function after stroke. *J. Neuroeng. Rehabil.* **2020**, *17*, 83. [CrossRef]
27. Maranesi, E.; Riccardi, G.R.; Di Donna, V.; Di Rosa, M.; Fabbietti, P.; Luzi, R.; Pranno, L.; Lattanzio, F.; Bevilacqua, R. Effectiveness of Intervention Based on End- effector Gait Trainer in Older Patients with Stroke: A Systematic Review. *J. Am. Med. Dir. Assoc.* **2020**, *21*, 1036–1044. [CrossRef]
28. Singh, H.; Unger, J.; Zariffa, J.; Pakosh, M.; Jaglal, S.; Craven, B.C.; Musselman, K.E. Robot-assisted upper extremity rehabilitation for cervical spinal cord injuries: A systematic scoping review. *Disabil. Rehabil. Assist. Technol.* **2018**, *13*, 704–715. [CrossRef]
29. Molteni, F.; Gasperini, G.; Cannaviello, G.; Guanziroli, E. Exoskeleton and End-Effector Robots for Upper and Lower Limbs Rehabilitation: Narrative Review. *PMR* **2018**, *10* (Suppl. S2), S174–S188. [CrossRef]
30. Lennon, O.; Tonellato, M.; Del Felice, A.; Di Marco, R.; Fingleton, C.; Korik, A.; Guanziroli, E.; Molteni, F.; Guger, C.; Otner, R.; et al. A Systematic Review Establishing the Current State-of-the-Art, the Limitations, and the DESIRED Checklist in Studies of Direct Neural Interfacing with Robotic Gait Devices in Stroke Rehabilitation. *Front. Neurosci.* **2020**, *14*, 578. [CrossRef]
31. Hobbs, B.; Artemiadis, P. A Review of Robot-Assisted Lower-Limb Stroke Therapy: Unexplored Paths and Future Directions in Gait Rehabilitation. *Front. Neurorobot.* **2020**, *15*, 14–19. [CrossRef] [PubMed]
32. Sheridan, T.B. A review of recent research in social robotics. *Curr. Opin. Psychol.* **2020**, *36*, 7–12. [CrossRef] [PubMed]
33. Uluer, P.; Kose, H.; Gumuslu, E.; Barkana, D.E. Experience with an Affective Robot Assistant for Children with Hearing Disabilities. *Int. J. Soc. Robot.* **2021**. [CrossRef] [PubMed]
34. Cobo Hurtado, L.; Viñas, P.F.; Zalama, E.; Gómez-García-Bermejo, J.; Delgado, J.M.; Vielba García, B. Development and Usability Validation of a Social Robot Platform for Physical and Cognitive Stimulation in Elder Care Facilities. *Healthcare* **2021**, *9*, 1067. [CrossRef]
35. Wudarczyk, O.A.; Kirtay, M.; Pischedda, D.; Hafner, V.V.; Haynes, J.D.; Kuhlen, A.K.; Abdel Rahman, R. Robots facilitate human language production. *Sci. Rep.* **2021**, *11*, 16737. [CrossRef]
36. Rietz, F.; SutherlanBensch, S.; Wermter, S.; Hellström, T. WoZ4U: An Open-Source Wizard-of-Oz Interface for Easy, Efficient and Robust HRI Experiments. *Front. Robot. AI* **2021**, *8*, 668057. [CrossRef]
37. Khan, Z.H.; Siddique, A.; Lee, C.W. Robotics Utilization for Healthcare Digitization in Global COVID-19 Management. *Int. J. Environ. Res. Public Health* **2020**, *17*, 3819. [CrossRef]
38. The Strong Robot with the Gentle Touch. Available online: https://www.riken.jp/en/news_pubs/research_news/pr/2015/20150223_2/ (accessed on 2 November 2021).
39. Gordon, J.S. Building Moral Robots: Ethical Pitfalls and Challenges. *Sci. Eng. Ethics.* **2020**, *26*, 141–157. [CrossRef]
40. Moor, J.H. The nature, importance, and difficulty of machine ethics. *Res. Gate* **2006**, *21*, 18–21. [CrossRef]
41. Lin, P.; Abney, K.; Bekey, G.A. (Eds.) Robot ethics: The Ethical and Social Implications of Robotics. In *Intelligent Robotics and Autonomous Agents*; MIT Press: Cambridge, MA, USA, 2014.
42. Wallach, W.; Allen, C. *Moral Machines: Teaching Robots Right from Wrong*; Oxford University Press: Oxford, UK, 2010.
43. Anderson, M.; Anderson, S.L. *Machine Ethics*; Cambridge University Press: Cambridge, MA, USA, 2011.
44. Gunkel, D.J.; Bryson, J. The machine as moral agent and patient. *Philos. Technol.* **2014**, *27*, 5–142. [CrossRef]

45. Available online: https://www.cambridge.org/core/books/machine-ethics/D7992C92BD465B54CA0D91871398AE5A (accessed on 2 November 2021).
46. Lennartz, S.; Dratsch, T.; Zopfs, D.; Persigehl, T.; Maintz, D.; Hokamp, N.G.; dos Santos, D.P. Use and Control of Artificial Intelligence in Patients Across the Medical Workflow: Single-Center Questionnaire Study of Patient Perspectives. *J. Med. Internet Res.* **2021**, *23*, e24221. [CrossRef]
47. Zhang, Z.; Citardi, D.; Wang, D.; Genc, Y.; Shan, J.; Fan, X. Patients' perceptions of using artificial intelligence (AI)-based technology to comprehend radiology imaging data. *Health Inform. J.* **2021**, *27*. [CrossRef]
48. Ongena, Y.P.; Haan, M.; Yakar, D.; Kwee, T.C. Patients' views on the implementation of artificial intelligence in radiology: Development and validation of a standardized questionnaire. *Eur. Radiol.* **2020**, *30*, 1033–1040. [CrossRef]
49. Hendrix, N.; Hauber, B.; Lee, C.I.; Bansal, A.; Veenstra, D.L. Artificial intelligence in breast cancer screening: Primary care provider preferences. *J. Am. Med. Inform. Assoc.* **2021**, *28*, 1117–1124. [CrossRef]
50. Abuzaid, M.M.; Elshami, W.; McConnell, J.; Tekin, H.O. An extensive survey oradiographers from the Middle East and India on artificial intelligence integration in radiology practice. *Health Technol.* **2021**, 1–6. [CrossRef]
51. Abuzaid, M.M.; Tekin, H.O.; Reza, M.; Elhag, I.R.; Elshami, W. Assessment of MRI technologists in acceptance and willingness to integrate artificial intelligence into practice. *Radiography* **2021**, *27* (Suppl S1), S83–S87. [CrossRef]
52. Giansanti, D.; Rossi, I.; Monoscalco, L. Lessons from the COVID-19 Pandemic on the Use of Artificial Intelligence in Digital Radiology: The Submission of a Survey to Investigate the Opinion of Insiders. *Healthcare* **2021**, *9*, 331. [CrossRef] [PubMed]
53. Abuzaid, M.M.; Elshami, W.; Tekin, H.; Issa, B. Assessment of the Willingness of Radiologists and Radiographers to Accept the Integration of Artificial Intelligence into Radiology Practice. *Acad. Radiol.* **2020**, *29*, 87–94. [CrossRef]
54. Alelyani, M.; Alamri, S.; Alqahtani, M.S.; Musa, A.; Almater, H.; Alqahtani, N.; Alshahrani, F.; Alelyani, S. Radiology Community Attitude in Saudi Arabia about the Applications of Artificial Intelligence in Radiology. *Healthcare* **2021**, *9*, 834. [CrossRef]
55. European Society of Radiology (ESR). Impact of artificial intelligence on radiology: A EuroAIM survey among members of the European Society of Radiology. *Insights Imaging* **2019**, *10*, 105. [CrossRef]
56. Galán, G.C.; Portero, F.S. Percepciones de estudiantes de Medicina sobre el impacto de la inteligencia artificial en radiología. *Radiología* **2021**. [CrossRef]
57. Available online: https://onlinelibrary.wiley.com/doi/abs/10.1002/9781118715598.ch20 (accessed on 2 November 2021).
58. Maccioni, G.; Giansanti, D. Medical Apps and the Gray Zone in the COVID-19 Era: Between Evidence and New Needs for Cybersecurity Expansion. *Healthcare* **2021**, *9*, 430. [CrossRef] [PubMed]
59. Lee, A.C. COVID-19 and the Advancement of Digital Physical Therapist Practice and Telehealth. *Phys. Ther.* **2020**, *100*, 1054–1057. [CrossRef] [PubMed]
60. Available online: https://pubmed.ncbi.nlm.nih.gov/?term=%28cybersecurity%29+AND+%28healthcare%29&sort=date&size=200 (accessed on 2 November 2021).
61. Available online: https://pubmed.ncbi.nlm.nih.gov/?term=%28cybersecurity%29+AND+%28healthcare%29+AND+%28care+robots%29&size=200 (accessed on 2 November 2021).
62. Stahl, B.C.; Coeckelbergh, M. Ethics of healthcare robotics: Towards responsible research and innovation. *Robot. Auton. Syst.* **2016**, *86*, 152–161. [CrossRef]
63. Coeckelbergh, M. Human development or human enhancement? A methodological reflection on capabilities and the evaluation of information technologies. *Ethics Inf. Technol.* **2011**, *13*, 81–92. [CrossRef]
64. Coeckelbergh, M. Are emotional robots deceptive? *IEEE Trans. Affective Comput.* **2012**, *3*, 388–393. [CrossRef]
65. Coeckelbergh, M. E-care as craftsmanship: Virtuous work, skilled engagement, and information technology in health care. *Med. Health Care Philos.* **2013**, *16*, 807–816. [CrossRef]
66. Coeckelbergh, M. Good Healthcare is in the "How": The Quality of Care, the Role of Machines, and the Need for New Skills. In *Machine Medical Ethics*; van Rysewyk, S.P., Pontier, M., Eds.; Springer: Berlin/Heidelberg, Germany, 2015; pp. 33–48.
67. Decker, M.; Fleischer, T. Contacting the brain—Aspects of a technology assessment of neural implants. *Biotechnol. J.* **2008**, *3*, 1502–1510. [CrossRef]
68. Sharkey, A.; Sharkey, N. Granny and the robots: Ethical issues in robot care for the elderly. *Ethics Inform. Technol.* **2010**, *14*, 27–40. [CrossRef]
69. Sparrow, R.; Sparrow, L. In the hands of machines? The future of aged care. *Minds Mach.* **2006**, *16*, 141–161. [CrossRef]
70. Whitby, B. Do you Want a Robot Lover? In *Robot Ethics: The Ethical and Social Implications of Robotics*; Lin, P., Abney, K., Bekey, G.A., Eds.; MIT Press: Cambridge, MA, USA, 2011; pp. 233–249.
71. McGlynn, E.A.; Kosecoff, J.; Brook, R.H. Format and conduct of consensus development conferences. Multi-nation comparison. *Int. J. Technol. Assess Health Care* **1990**, *6*, 450–469. [CrossRef]
72. d'Accréditation, A.N. d'Evaluation en Santé: Les Conférences de Consensus. In *Base Méthodologique Pour Leur Réalisation en France*; ANAES: Paris, France, 1999.
73. Candiani, G.; Colombo, C.; Daghini, R.; Magrini, N.; Mosconi, P.; Nonino, F.; Satolli, R.; Come Organizzare una Conferenza di Consenso. Manuale Metodologico, Roma, ISS-SNLG. Available online: https://www.psy.it/wp-content/uploads/2018/02/Manuale-Metodologico-Consensus.pdf (accessed on 2 November 2021).

74. Arcelloni, M.C.; Broggi, F.; Cortese, S.; Della Corte, G.; Pirozzolo, V.; Consensus Conference: Uno Strumento Per La Pratica Clinica. Riferimenti Storico-Metodologici e Stato dell'arte dei Lavori Italiani sul Disturbo Primario del Linguaggio e sui Disturbi Specifici dell'Apprendimento. 2009. Available online: https://rivistedigitali.erickson.it/il-tnpee/archivio/vol-1-n-1/riferimenti-storico-metodologici-e-stato-dellarte-dei-lavori-italiani-sul-disturbo-primario-del-linguaggio-e-sui-disturbi-specifici-dellapprendimento/ (accessed on 2 November 2021).
75. Available online: https://springerhealthcare.it/mr/archivio/la-conferenza-italiana-di-consenso-sulla-robotica-in-riabilitazione/ (accessed on 2 November 2021).
76. Boldrini, P.; Bonaiuti, D.; Mazzoleni, S.; Posteraro, F. Rehabilitation assisted by robotic and electromechanical devices for people with neurological disabilities: Contributions for the preparation of a national conference in Italy. *Eur. J. Phys. Rehabil. Med.* **2021**, *57*, 458–459. [CrossRef]
77. Available online: https://2020.hci.international/files/HCII2020_Final_Program.pdf (accessed on 2 November 2021).
78. Coventry, L.; Branley-Bell, D.; Sillence, E.; Magalini, S.; Mari, P.; Magkanaraki, A.; Anastasopoulou, K. Cyber-Risk in Healthcare: Exploring Facilitators and Barriers to Secure Behaviour. In Proceedings of the 22nd International Conference on Human Computer Interaction, Copenhagen, Denmark, 19–24 July 2020; pp. 105–122.
79. Dolic, Z.; Castro, R.; Moarcas, A.; Robots in Healthcare: A Solution or a Problem? Study for the Committee on Environment, Public Health, and Food Safety. Luxembourg: Policy Department for Economic, Scientific and Quality of Life Policies, European Parli Ment; 2019. Available online: https://www.europarl.europa.eu/RegData/etudes/IDAN/2019/638391/IPOL_IDA (accessed on 2 November 2021).

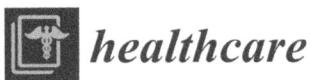

Viewpoint

The Cybersecurity and the Care Robots: A Viewpoint on the Open Problems and the Perspectives

Daniele Giansanti [1,*] **and Rosario Alfio Gulino** [2]

[1] Centre Tisp, Istituto Superiore di Sanità, 00161 Rome, Italy
[2] Faculty of Engineering, Tor Vergata University, Via Cracovia, 00133 Roma, Italy; rosario.gulino.uni.tv@hotmail.com
* Correspondence: daniele.giansanti@iss.it; Tel.: +39-06-49902701

Abstract: Care robots represent an opportunity for the health domain. The use of these robots has important implications. They can be used in surgery, rehabilitation, assistance, therapy, and other medical fields. Therefore, care robots (CR)s, have both important physical and psychological implications during their use. Furthermore, these devices, meet important data in clinical applications. These data must be protected. Therefore, cybersecurity (CS) has become a crucial characteristic that concerns all the involved actors. The study investigated the collocation of CRs in the context of CS studies in the health domain. Problems and peculiarities of these devices, with reference to the CS, were faced, investigating in different scientific databases. Highlights, ranging also from ethics implications up to the regulatory legal framework (ensuring safety and cybersecurity) have been reported. Models and cyber-attacks applicable on the CRs have been identified.

Keywords: e-health; medical devices; m-health; rehabilitation; robotics; organization models; artificial intelligence; electronic surveys; social robots; collaborative robots; cyber security; cyber risk; informatics

Citation: Giansanti, D.; Gulino, R.A. The Cybersecurity and the Care Robots: A Viewpoint on the Open Problems and the Perspectives. *Healthcare* **2021**, *9*, 1653. https://doi.org/10.3390/healthcare9121653

Academic Editor: Tin-Chih Toly Chen

Received: 5 November 2021
Accepted: 24 November 2021
Published: 29 November 2021

Publisher's Note: MDPI stays neutral with regard to jurisdictional claims in published maps and institutional affiliations.

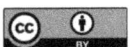

Copyright: © 2021 by the authors. Licensee MDPI, Basel, Switzerland. This article is an open access article distributed under the terms and conditions of the Creative Commons Attribution (CC BY) license (https://creativecommons.org/licenses/by/4.0/).

1. Introduction

The cybersecurity (CS) in healthcare deals with the cyber risks in the cyber-systems used in the *health domain*. These systems can be medical devices and/or a complex interoperable and heterogeneous systems (e.g., Radiology Information System) [1,2]. A frightening growth is expected in the sector of the care robots (CR)s. The applications of social robots [3,4], for example, are continuously increasing [5,6].

Hence, it is now very important to address CS in CRs.

The Policy Department for Economic, Scientific and Quality of Life Policies, of the European Parliament, identified the most interesting applications for the CRs [7]: *Robotic surgery, Care and Socially assistive Robots, Rehabilitation systems, Training for health and care workers*. The sector is wide, complex and with numerous implications for the CS. For example, the rehabilitation robotics [8] has three motion applications (Table 1):

1. The stability.
2. The lower limbs.
3. The upper limbs.

Furthermore, rehabilitation robots use two different technological solutions (exoskeleton technology and end-effector technology), with different implications for the CS.

Social robots (SR)s are used in several diversified fields of assistance and rehabilitation [3,4]. Similar considerations can be carried out for the other applications. The implications between technologies, applications and CS immediately emerge from the definition of CR. CRs are complex and interoperable systems [9]. The European Foresight Monitoring Network [10] defines the CR as a system "able to perform coordinated mechatronic actions (force or movement exertions) based on processing information acquired through sensor technology, to support the functioning of impaired individuals, medical interventions, care and rehabilitation of patients and also individuals in prevention programs".

Table 1. Classification of the rehabilitation robot according to the applications.

Application	Description
Upper limb rehabilitation	Allowing rehabilitation of the upper limb using exoskeletons or end-effector system
Lower limb rehabilitation	Allowing rehabilitation of the lower limb using exoskeletons or end-effector system
Stability	Allowing the stability training and recovery using exoskeletons or end-effector system

The European Parliament traced for the CR the direction of the CS, highlighting that (literally cited) "possible applications of AI and robotics in medical care (are) managing medical records and data, performing repetitive jobs (analysing tests, X-rays, CT scans, data entry), treatment design, digital consultation (such as medical consultation based on personal medical history and common medical knowledge), virtual nurses, medication management, drug creation, precision medicine (as genetics and genomics look for mutations and links to disease from the information in DNA), health monitoring and healthcare system analysis, among other." [11].

It is important to investigate the progress of CS studies on the CRs. It is also important to investigate the problems and peculiarities. Correlations with other disciplines are important, such as, for example, ethics and regulation.

CRs, in fact, have characteristics, that are not found on other devices. They can replace caregivers or provide psychological or motor rehabilitation. The implications of CS in a programming error or a sabotage are high. Traditional problems can be found. However, many others are added. Motor damage can occur. Psychological damage can occur. Think about the false relationship that can be created with a pet SR. Think about the problems that an incorrect programming of the ethics concepts of an SR can bring.

The objective of the study is:
(a) To investigate the positioning of CRs in CS studies.
(b) Analyse the problems and peculiarities of the devices that have an impact in this area.
(c) Take stock of the related issues of ethics and regulation.

In this paper the authors discuss the conception of a viewpoint, presented and explained in four sections (plus the introduction and conclusions).

The first section (paragraph 2: The position of the care robots in the studies) deals with the state of production of studies in this area. This is carried out through an analysis of the production of scientific literature. The second section (paragraph 3: Ethics, care robots and cybersecurity) deals with the impact of the ethical issues. In particular, the correlation of the CS both with the ethics of research and with the programming of ethics on CRs is highlighted. The third section (paragraph 4: Regulatory framework, care robots and cybersecurity) deals with the situation of the regulatory framework. The fourth section (paragraph 5: Cyber-attacks applicable to care robots) reports models and cyber-attacks.

2. The Position of the Care Robots in the Studies

We are certainly witnessing a growing interest in the CS.

A simple search on the Pubmed database, the most important database of the health domain, shows 12.785 results on the cyber security [12]. Among them, a group identified in [13] deals with robots. By expanding the search with the keys safety and risk we find:

4882 articles with the key (safety [Title/Abstract]) AND (robot) [14].

5005 articles with the key (risk [Title/Abstract]) AND (robot) [15].

Scientists refer to safety or risk also to address issues related to informatic faults/problems. These informatic problems/faults can affect the mechatronics, and therefore, the human interface. This is a CS issue. Certainly, this is a first important indication for scholars. The experience gained in the sector in the industry, production, and consuming sector (IPCS) is another important issue to consider. Here, the theme of the safety of robot-human interaction in the workplace is highly developed. Here, the topic has been dealt with for much longer. Safety in robots is addressed. However, the use of robots for security is also addressed. Both are CS related issues. Part of the experience gained here, can be exported and readapted in the health domain, a particular workplace. Presently [16], there are three categories of robots in the IPCS: (1) industrial robots; (2) professional and personal service robots, and (3) collaborative robots. Studies reporting recommendations are spreading for these types of robots [16,17]. Some studies are specifically dealing with physical security [18] also in relation to CS. Other studies are dealing with traditional issues, such as security and privacy issues [19].

Very interesting models dealt with the security in the workplace. The Advanced Human-Robot Collaboration Model (AHRCM) approach was proposed in [20]. The idea was to enhance the risk assessment and to improve the safety in the workplace. The experimental results showed that the proposed AHRCM model achieved high performance in human-robot collaboration to reduce the risk.

The recent review in [21] highlighted how CS experience in IPCS robotics is exportable to the world of CRs. The same authors highlighted models and types of cyber-attacks on the CRs. Recent studies dealt with the security with SRs [22]. This included: risk assessment of communications security, predictive analysis of security risks, implementing access control policies to enhance the security of solution, and auditing of the solution against security, safety and privacy guidelines and regulations. A limited approach to some issues of CS was addressed in a few studies, such as in surgical applications [23] or in the rehabilitation of the lower limbs [24].

Other studies showed a backwardness in importing into the health domain the experience made elsewhere [25]. Probably, this is due to the limits and inadequacy of legislation concerning the CS [9,26]. It is also very important to observe how scientific societies move around the CS theme.

For example, CS has now become an indispensable issue in the topic Human Computer Interaction (HCI), in international scientific meetings [27]. In fact, one of the most important international conferences on HCI, hosts a section (HCI-CPT: International Conference on HCI for Cybersecurity, Privacy and Trust) dedicated to the CS applied to HCI. This highlights the importance of the theme for machines that interface/integrate with the human. In [28], a work presented at the HCI-CPT, it is also highlighted how the analysis must be extended directly in the field (for example in the workplace), involving the insiders in targeted investigations, with dedicated surveys, to understand behaviours at risk, as regards CS.

It is also necessary to consider the peculiarities of the CRs.

The ethical implications for the CRs are much more relevant than for other categories of robots. It is also necessary to consider more risks and criticalities. These risks and criticalities affect not only the physical issues, but also the psychological issues [9].

It was proposed in [9] a model describing the relationships between cyber-attacks/software fault/AI deficit and the impact on human safety.

We specialize in Figure 1, the model in the case of rehabilitation and assistance robotics. This model highlights the health risks for the user.

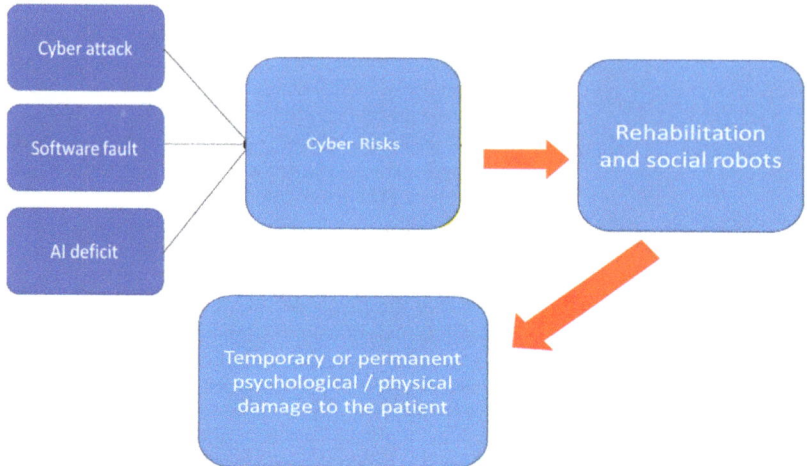

Figure 1. Model of health risks for the CRs.

3. Ethics, Care Robots and Cybersecurity

Very important ethical discussions are open. A search on Pubmed with the key (social robot) AND (ethics) shows some interesting scientific contributes [29], confirming the wide discussion around the ethics. Ethics has a strong impact on the world of the CRs. This is reflected in the CS. We extended here the search also to other databases.

We can undoubtedly distinguish two important macro-sectors with an impact on CS. The first macro-sector is the ethics in a responsible research and innovation [30]. The second macro-sector is the ethics problem encountered while building moral CRs [31].

Stahl and Coeckelbergh highlighted, for the first macro-sector [30], that traditional approaches to the ethics of robotics are often distant from innovation practices and contexts of use. They listed in their review key concerns of ethics. As it has been highlighted in [30] there is a strong scientific production of ethics of CRs [32–39], or machine (medical) ethics [40–44] connected to the CRs. Three aspects were identified in [30].

First, there are important impacts both in the society and in the health domain:
Replacement and its implications for labour.
Replacement and its implications for the quality of care; they are the so-called de-humanisation and "cold" care.

Second, there are issues raised by human–robot interaction in the health domain and especially by the robot taking over tasks from humans, for instance: autonomy (connected to the implication of the robots take decision with autonomy) Role and tasks (connected to the changes in the workflow), Responsibility (connected to the responsibility chain in case of problems), The Deception (connected, for example, to the use of SRs as 'social companions, related to questions of opportunities and justification). Trust (connected, for example, to the reliability of giving subjects (also frail) in the hands of a CR.

Third, there are issues traditionally connected to the CS as for example:
Privacy and data protection.
Safety and avoidance of harm.

The second macro-sector [31] on the ethics problems is encountered while building moral CRs. It focuses on the interdisciplinary field of machine ethics—that is, how to program ethical rules and concepts inside on a robot [45]. This sector has become of utmost importance because the recent technological developments in the field of the CRs and artificial intelligence in general [46–50]. Gordon highlighted that to make ethics [31] "computable" (literally cited "depends in part, on how the designers understand ethics and attempt to implement that understanding in programs, but also more generally on their expertise in the field".

Based on the review [31] it was found that, scholars in the field in informatics applied to machine ethics have gaps in training and practical knowledge of ethics. There is therefore an important CS due to this.

From the previous analysis, a strong connection emerges between ethical issues and CS in the CRs. There is a strong need to rethink a more expanded CS also connected to the ethics in robotics.

4. Regulatory Framework, Care Robots and Cybersecurity

Surely when we consider the regulatory issues, we must ponder that CRs also use eHealth [51]. However, many other issues must be considered [9,26]. These issues range from the impact of mechatronics up to the use as a networked medical device. Some studies have highlighted lights and shadows of the regulatory framework [9], arranged in Europe into:

- Safety regulations [52].
- Legislation on medical devices (MD)s classification [53].
- Legal frameworks on the cybersecurity [54,55].

4.1. Care Robots and Safety Regulations

Robots, in general, and CRs, follow [52] the General Product Safety Directive (Directive 2001/95/EC of the European Parliament and of the Council of 3 December 2001 on general product safety 2001) and the Directive 85/374/EEC on liability for defective products. The applicability of product liability regulations is not easily and directly applicable in the context of robotics applications.

4.2. Care Robots and Medical Device Regulation

CRs, based on their destination of use, can be classified as a medical device (MD). The European Medical Device Regulation (Regulation (EU) 2017/745) [53] contains a detailed definition of MDs.

The Regulation contains three important actions (lights) in the direction of the CS concerning the minimization of the risks, the design of the software (including CS), the inclusion of the respect of a set of IT requirements also related to the CS.

The regulation [53] certainly presents great innovations for the CS. However, there are some shadows. The first shadow is that this regulation focuses a lot on manufacturers and little on recipients/users [9,26], who have a leading role. Perhaps, instruction sheets and manuals are not always enough. The second shadow [9,26] is that compliance with CS requirements is challenging, in part due to the potential overlap of different certification schemes with varying geographical or product scope and evolution of external regulations (see for example the Cybersecurity Act). The third shadow, we personally think applicable is that the intended use and certification must be aligned [8] and this it is not always easy to detect.

4.3. Care Robots and Regulations on the Cybersecurity

Three are the documents regarding the legal frameworks regulating CR CS [54–56]:

1. The directive on security of network and information systems (also called NIS Directive) that provides measures for boosting the overall CS in the EU [54].
2. The General Data Protection Regulation (GDPR) obligating to implement appropriate measures to ensure a level of security appropriate to relevant risks [55].
3. The EU Cyber-security Act (Regulation (EU) 2019/881) which establishes an EU-wide cybersecurity certification framework [57].

None of the documents has been specifically designed for CRs.
The first two documents [53,54] work in synergy.

According to the NIS Directive, operators need to respond appropriately to manage the CS in a network [9]. A Network can, (according to the NIS Directive [54]), include MDs, such as robots. As the healthcare providers also process personal data, they are, therefore, subject to the provisions of the GDPR [55].

The third document, the EU cybersecurity Act establishes a road map for voluntary CS certifications valid in the EU [56].

Among the evident limitations of the three documents [54–56] (in addition to the fact that they are not specifically designed for CRs) we find that: the first two delegate CS to healthcare providers, although they can be found on the market CRs with very different levels of CS [9]. The third document provides for a certification, but this is only voluntary.

5. Cyber-Attacks Applicable to Care Robots

CS for CRs must consider a broader spectrum of problems than other critical MDs, where, nevertheless, CS is more consolidated, such as the pacemakers [57–59] and the artificial pancreas [60–62]. CRs can generate, for example a psychological harm (Figure 1). This is also a consequence of issues dealt in par. 3 [30,31]. Much of the experience in robotics [16–20] on physiological harms/damages can be exported to CRs. Indeed, in [21] a process of unification has been carried out, which has general validity. Figure 2 summarizes the different robot-related threats, their causes, and their consequences in the case of the CRs. With reference to the figure, the nature of the attack is: internal vs external, coordinated vs random, detected/undetected, corrected/uncorrected. The identification is: data confidentiality and privacy, message authentication, device/user authentication, system integrity, data availability, system availability. The target is: the application layer, the hardware layer, the firmware layer. The impact can be low, moderate, high. The trust and safety concerns (according to the model in paragraph 2) are data integrity and privacy, physical harm, physical damage, psychological harm.

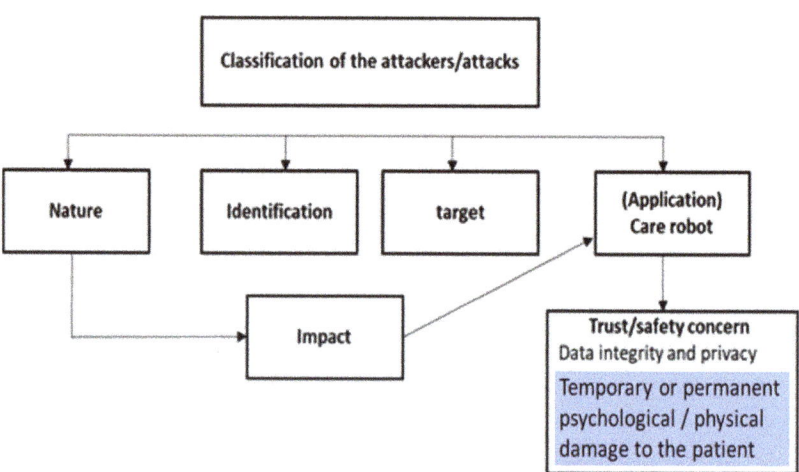

Figure 2. Model of robot-related threats, causes, and consequences.

The Attacks can be arranged into three categories [21]: ATTACKs on the hardware, ATTACKs on firmware, ATTACKs on the communication. In the following, we summarize these categories in brief.

5.1. Attacks on the Hardware

These ATTACKs [21] vary from hardware Trojans up to phishing [63]. They allow the aggressor to create passages to gain unauthorized access up a full control [21,64]. In some cases, they can even have a full access to the hardware. We can also find the implementation ATTACKs or fault ATTACKs [64]. These are very dangerous and can cause to sensitive data damage or system corruption.

5.2. Attacks on the Firmware

According to [21,65,66], as the OS upgrading/maintenance is mainly performed using the internet, the OS is exposed to DoS and D-DoS ATTACKs, along with the indiscriminate programme execution, and root-kit ATTACKs. Furthermore, the Applications in the CRs, are vulnerable to application ATTACKs. These ATTACKs comprehend malware, worms, viruses, software Trojans ATTACKs, buffer overflow, and malicious code injection ATTACKs [67]. Figure 3 reports examples of these ATTACKs [21,67–73]:

Worm attacks. ATTACKs that aim to target the robotic systems by exploiting the vulnerabilities of their network's connected devices [67].

Ransomware attacks. ATTACKs that aim to encrypt all the data linked to robotic systems, devices, and applications [68].

Trojans and random access trojan ATTACKs. These ATTACKs are usually masqueraded in the form of a legitimate application and sometimes can be carried out via a phishing email or in a form of a Winlocker.

Rootkit attacks. These ATTACKs allow a given attacker to have a privileged controlled access on an administrator level with the ability to have access to information and data related to robots and robotic systems.

Botnet attacks. These ATTACKs are usually employed as bots to conduct D-DoS attacks against medical systems. Botnets can be based on malicious codes used to infect unprotected robotic devices.

Spyware attacks. The purpose of these ATTACKs is to gather information and data about the robot operator, the connected device, and the robot in use, to send this information to malicious third party.

Buffer overflow attacks. They aim to exploit the system vulnerability to manipulate a robotics' device memory to control the robot and hijack it.

Password cracking. ATTACKs with the aim to target the authentication of the robotic systems, to gain a full access privilege [69].

Reverse engineering attacks. These ATTACKs are also known as a person-to-person ATTACKs. They aim to convince their victim(s) that they are legitimate users

Surveillance attacks. These ATTACKs include creating malicious robotic applications, third-party applications and anti-virus systems masqueraded as legitimate ones and include also fake updates and pop-ups that urges robotic users from clicking on them to fulfil the update task.

Malicious code injection (MCI) attacks or Remote Code Execution (RCE) attacks. They are based on an attacker's capability of executing malicious codes to perform an injection attack [70-71].

Phishing attacks. They are still ongoing with a variety of phishing ATTACK types [72-73] targeting robotic employees and firms with different privileges and access level.

Figure 3. Examples of ATTACKs on the firmware.

5.3. Attacks on Communications

Robotic communications are also exposed to different ATTACKs [21,74–77] that can affect different levels of security at different levels of communication (Figure 4):

Jamming attacks. They have the aim to interrupt and disrupt the robot-to-robot and robot-to-humans communication.
De-authentication attacks. They aim to disable the robotic devices temporarily or periodically from being able to connect back to their initial operator, disrupting the communication.
Traffic analysis attacks They aim to listen the ongoing traffic between the robots and the human actors.
Eavesdropping attacks. They aim to passively monitor the transmitted robotic traffic over encrypted and unencrypted open communication channels.
False data injection attacks. These ATTACKs have as target the privacy and integrity of the robotic data and the availability of robots, by intercepting and modifying its payload [74].
(Distributed) denial of service attacks. They aim to prevent legitimate users from accessing robotic systems and devices. DoS ATTACKs, for example, send excessive requests, that lead the network to continuously re-authenticate requests having invalid return addresses [75].
Replay attacks. They occur when a given adversary stores and replays, later, the old messages sent between the robot and its operator to disrupt the ongoing traffic.
Masquerading attacks. This ATTACK masquerade a valid identity. The attacker, therefore, seems to be authentic. This attack has different objectives such as slowing down or up the speed of a robot, which may lead to an incident, or target its operational activity and performance.
Man-in-the-Middle (MiMA) attacks. These ATTACKs aim to listen and intercept the communication between two robotic systems, alter the information and inject it without being detected [76].
Meet-in-the-Middle (MITM) attacks. These ATTACKs aim to break the encrypted communication channel and either actively or passively eavesdrop.
Identity attacks. This type of ATTACKs includes, for example the identity revealing ATTACKs
Network impersonation attacks. They aim to obtain the credentials of a legitimate entity in a given robotic network by claiming its network ID.
Message tampering-fabrication-alteration attacks. These ATTACKs aim to alter the integrity of the exchanged messages, for example creating fake messages.
Illusion attacks. They are ATTACKs are placed in the network to generate false data. As a result, false data can spread over the network.

ATTACKs On Communication

Figure 4. Examples of ATTACKs on the communication.

6. Conclusions
6.1. Highlights

CRs [7] represent an opportunity for the health domain. The use of these robots has important implications. They can be used in surgery [7], in important and delicate clinical interventions both in presence and in tele-surgery. They can be used on frail patients, in rehabilitation processes [8]. They can be used in psychological and cognitive rehabilitation processes, as in the case of SRs, in children, elderly, and other subjects with disabilities [3,4]. Therefore, they have important physical and psychological implications during their use [9]. Furthermore, these devices, during their use, encounter important demographic-and-clinical data and other reserved information; all data that must be protected, in accordance with current regulations [1,2]. CS has consequently become a crucial issue. It concerns all the actors involved (from the design process to its use; from the manufacturer up to the patient and the caregiver). The study investigated the collocation of CRs in the context of CS studies in the health domain, also in comparison to other sectors. Problems and peculiarities were faced, investigating in different scientific database. They ranged from ethics and safety up to legislation and regulation issues.

The highlights of the study are as follows:

- A simple search on the Pubmed database, the most important database of the health domain, shows 12.785 results on the CS [12]. Among these, an important group [13] is dedicated to robotics. However, many studies on robotics linked to CS can be traced with the other keys safety and risk [14,15].
- CRs have peculiarities that make them unique. However, regarding some issues, the experience of robotics used in the IPCS robotics can be partly taken into consideration [16–20].

- CRs are complex mechatronic tools, but also HCI and devices integrated to eHealth [27,28,51]. Scientific support come also from both initiatives of scientific societies, operating in these sectors [27] and proper approaches on the insiders [28].
- Ethics has an important role and a peculiarity on CRs, such as on the SRs [29]. An in-depth analysis of the ethical issues in this discipline has identified two macro-sectors [30,31]. The first macro-sector is the ethics in a responsible research and innovation [30]. The second macro-sector is the ethics problem encountered while building moral CRs [31]. A strong connection emerges between ethical issues and CS from the examination of the two macro-sectors (also correlated). There is a strong need to rethink a CS connected to ethics issues.
- The models between the Cyber ATTACKs/ Software default/AI deficits and the physical/ psychological impact, have been identified [9]. They also embed the problems identified in the previous point [30,31]. These models show a wider range of CS problems than other consolidated MDs [57–62].
- Cyber ATTACKs applicable on the CRs, and the related impact, have been identified and categorized into three groups [21] concerning hardware [63,64], firmware [65–73], and communication [74–77].
- Targeted surveys with interviews and questionnaires regarding the CS behaviours of insiders with CRs will have to be conducted, as already been carried out, for example, in the health domain generally [28]. This will be useful for building medical knowledge.
- There are shadows in EU MD regulations [53]. First, it focuses a lot on manufacturers and little on recipients/ users. Second, [9] the compliance with CS requirements is challenging, in part due to the potential overlap of different certification schemes with varying geographical or product scope and evolution of external to the MDR regulations. Third, the intended use and certification, often, do not seem aligned.
- There are limits in the application of specific CS certifications. They are voluntary, as in the case of the Cybersecurity ACT [56].
- The CRs would need an ad hoc regulatory framework, in consideration of the peculiarities.

6.2. Reflections

We believe that, in the light of what is covered in our study, it is important to plan an acculturalization process on CS, with specific reference to CRs. This process must concern all the involved actors, from the builders up to the users, and the caregivers. It must be conducted in the different environments (e.g., home and the hospital). Training in this area must become an important issue. In addition, agreement initiatives (e.g., guidelines, consensus conferences, and technology assessment initiative [78–84]) considering CS could be welcome. Stakeholders will have to take actions in this area, through consensus initiatives (for example, considering the CS in consensus conferences), specific monitoring initiatives (for example through targeted surveys), and specific interventions on the training.

Author Contributions: Conceptualization, D.G.; methodology, D.G.; software, D.G., R.A.G.; validation, D.G., R.A.G.; formal analysis, D.G.; investigation, D.G.; resources, D.G., R.A.G.; data curation, D.G.; writing—original draft preparation, D.G.; writing—review and editing, All; visualization, All; supervision, All; project administration, D.G. All authors have read and agreed to the published version of the manuscript.

Funding: This research received no external funding.

Institutional Review Board Statement: Not applicable.

Informed Consent Statement: Not applicable.

Data Availability Statement: Not applicable.

Conflicts of Interest: The authors declare no conflict of interest.

References

1. Giansanti, D. Cybersecurity and the digital-health: The challenge of this millennium. *Healthcare* **2021**, *9*, 62. [CrossRef]
2. Giansanti, D.; Monoscalco, L. The cyber-risk in cardiology: Towards an investigation on the self-perception among the cardiologists. *Mhealth* **2021**, *7*, 28. [CrossRef]
3. Cobo Hurtado, L.; Viñas, P.F.; Zalama, E.; Gómez-GarcíaBermejo, J.; Delgado, J.M.; Vielba García, B. Development and usability validation of a social robot platform for physical and cognitive stimulation in elder care facilities. *Healthcare* **2021**, *9*, 1067. [CrossRef]
4. Sheridan, T.B. A review of recent research in social robotics. *Curr. Opin. Psychol.* **2020**, *36*, 7–12.
5. Mejia, C.; Kajikawa, Y. Bibliometric analysis of social robotics research: Identifying research trends and knowledgebase. *Appl. Sci.* **2017**, *7*, 1316.
6. Social Robots Market—Growth, Trends, COVID-19 Impact, and Forecasts (2021–2026). Available online: https://www.mordorintelligence.com/industry-reports/social-robots-market (accessed on 22 February 2021).
7. Dolic, Z.; Castro, R.; Moarcas, A. Robots in Healthcare: A Solution or a Problem? Study for the Committee on Environment, Public Health, and Food Safety. Luxembourg: Policy Department for Economic, Scientific and Quality of Life Policies, European Parliament. 2019. Available online: https://www.europarl.europa.eu/RegData/etudes/IDAN/2019/638391/IPOL_IDA(2019)638391_EN.pdf (accessed on 25 November 2021).
8. Boldrini, P.; Bonaiuti, D.; Mazzoleni, S.; Posteraro, F. Rehabilitation assisted by robotic and electromechanical devices for people with neurological disabilities: Contributions for the preparation of a national conference in Italy. *Eur. J. Phys. Rehabil. Med.* **2021**, *57*, 458–459. [CrossRef]
9. Fosch-Villaronga, E.; Mahler, T. Safety and robots: Strengthening the link between cybersecurity and safety in the context of care robots. *Comput. Law Secur. Rev.* **2021**, *41*, 105528.
10. European Foresight Monitoring Network, EFMN (2008) Roadmap Robotics for Healthcare. Foresight Brief No. 157. Available online: http://www.foresight-platform.eu/wp-content/uploads/2011/02/EFMN-Brief-No.-157_Robotics-for-Healthcare.pdf (accessed on 22 February 2021).
11. European Parliament Resolution of 12 February 2019 on a Comprehensive European Industrial Policy on Artificial Intelligence and Robotics (2018/2088(INI)). Available online: http://www.europarl.europa.eu/doceo/document/TA-8-2019-0081_EN.pdf (accessed on 22 February 2021).
12. Specific Research on the Pubmed Database. Available online: https://pubmed.ncbi.nlm.nih.gov/?term=%28cybersecurity%29+AND+%28healthcare%29&sort=date&size=200 (accessed on 25 November 2021).
13. Specific Research on the Pubmed Database: (cybersecurity) AND (healthcare) AND (care robots). Available online: https://pubmed.ncbi.nlm.nih.gov/?term=%28cybersecurity%29+AND+%28healthcare%29+AND+%28care+robots%29&sort=date&size=200 (accessed on 25 November 2021).
14. Specific Research on the Pubmed Database: (safey[Title/Abstract]) AND (robot). Available online: https://pubmed.ncbi.nlm.nih.gov/?term=%28safey%5BTitle%2FAbstract%5D%29+AND+%28robot%29&sort=date (accessed on 25 November 2021).
15. Specific Research on the Pubmed Database: (risk [Title/Abstract]) AND (robot). Available online: https://pubmed.ncbi.nlm.nih.gov/?term=%28risk+%5BTitle%2FAbstract%5D%29+AND+%28robot%29&sort=date&size=200 (accessed on 22 November 2021).
16. Murashov, V.; Hearl, F.; Howard, J. Working safely with robot workers: Recommendations for the new workplace. *J. Occup. Environ. Hyg.* **2016**, *13*, D61–D71. [CrossRef]
17. Missala, T. Paradigms and safety requirements for a new generation of workplace equipment. *Int. J. Occup. Saf. Ergon.* **2014**, *20*, 249–256. [CrossRef] [PubMed]
18. Bortot, D.; Ding, H.; Antonopolous, A.; Bengler, K. Human motion behavior while interacting with an industrial robot. *Work* **2012**, *41* (Suppl. 1), 1699–1707. [CrossRef]
19. Guangnan, Z.; Tao, H.; Rahman, M.A.; Yao, L.; Al-Saffar, A.; Meng, Q.; Liu, W.; Yaseen, Z.M. Security and privacy issues related to the workplace-based security robot system. *Work* **2021**, *68*, 871–879. [CrossRef]
20. Zheyuan, C.; Rahman, M.A.; Tao, H.; Liu, Y.; Pengxuan, D.; Yaseen, Z.M. Need for developing a security robot-based risk management for emerging practices in the workplace using the Advanced Human-Robot Co. *Work* **2021**, *68*, 1–10.
21. Yaacoub, J.A.; Noura, H.N.; Salman, O.; Chehab, A. Robotics cyber security: Vulnerabilities, attacks, countermeasures, and recommendations. *Int. J. Inf. Secur.* **2021**, *19*, 1–44. [CrossRef]
22. Vulpe, A.; Crăciunescu, R.; Drăgulinescu, A.M.; Kyriazakos, S.; Paikan, A.; Ziafati, P. Enabling security services in socially assistive robot scenarios for healthcare applications. *Sensors* **2021**, *21*, 6912. [CrossRef]
23. Liu, Y.; Yi, Y.; Deng, P.; Zhang, W. Preclinical evaluation of the new EDGE SP 1000 single-port robotic surgical system in gynecology minimal access surgery. *Surg. Endosc.* **2021**, 1–6, (Online ahead of print). [CrossRef]
24. Li, I.H.; Lin, Y.S.; Lee, L.W.; Lin, W.T. Design, manufacturing, and control of a pneumatic-driven passive robotic gait training system for muscle-weakness in a lower limb. *Sensors* **2021**, *21*, 6709. [CrossRef]
25. Lhotska, L. Application of industry 4.0 concept to health care. *Stud. Health Technol. Inform.* **2020**, *273*, 23–37. [CrossRef] [PubMed]
26. Jarota, M. Artificial intelligence and robotisation in the EU—should we change OHS law? *J. Occup. Med. Toxicol.* **2021**, *16*, 18. [CrossRef]
27. HCI 2020 International 22st International Conference on Human—Computer Interaction. Available online: https://2020.hci.international/files/HCII2020_Final_Program.pdf (accessed on 25 November 2021).

28. Coventry, L.; Branley-Bell, D.; Sillence, E.; Magalini, S.; Mari, P.; Magkanaraki, A.; Anastasopoulou, K. Cyber-risk in healthcare: Exploring facilitators and barriers to secure behaviour. In Proceedings of the 22nd International Conference on Human Computer Interaction, Copenhagen, Denmark, 19–24 July 2020; Springer: Berlin/Heidelberg, Germany, 2020; pp. 105–122.
29. Specific Research on the Pubmed Database: (social robot) AND (ethics). Available online: https://pubmed.ncbi.nlm.nih.gov/?term=%28social+robot%29+AND+%28ethics%29&sort=date&size=200 (accessed on 25 November 2021).
30. Stahl, B.C.; Coeckelbergh, M. Ethics of healthcare robotics: Towards responsible research and innovation. *Robot. Auton. Syst.* **2016**, *86*, 152–161.
31. Gordon, J.S. Building moral robots: Ethical pitfalls and challenges. *Sci. Eng. Ethics* **2020**, *26*, 141–157. [CrossRef]
32. Coeckelbergh, M. Human development or human enhancement? A methodological reflection on capabilities and the evaluation of information technologies. *Ethics Inf. Technol.* **2011**, *13*, 81–92. [CrossRef]
33. Coeckelbergh, M. Are emotional robots deceptive? *IEEE Trans. Affect. Comput.* **2012**, *3*, 388–393. [CrossRef]
34. Coeckelbergh, M. E-care as craftsmanship: Virtuous work, skilled engagement, and information technology in health care. *Med. Health Care Philos.* **2013**, *16*, 807–816.
35. Coeckelbergh, M. Good healthcare is in the "how": The quality of care, the role of machines, and the need for new skills. In *Machine Medical Ethics*; van Rysewyk, S.P., Pontier, M., Eds.; Springer: Berlin/Heidelberg, Germany, 2015; pp. 33–48.
36. Decker, M.; Fleischer, T. Contacting the brain—aspects of a technology assessment of neural implants. *Biotechnol. J.* **2008**, *3*, 1502–1510. [CrossRef]
37. Sharkey, A.; Sharkey, N. Granny and the robots: Ethical issues in robot care for the elderly. *Ethics Inform. Technol.* **2010**, *14*, 27–40.
38. Sparrow, R.; Sparrow, L. In the hands of machines? The future of aged care. *Minds Mach.* **2006**, *16*, 141–161.
39. Whitby, B. Do you want a robot lover. In *Robot Ethics: The Ethical and Social Implications of Robotics*; Lin, P., Abney, K., Bekey, G.A., Eds.; MIT Press: Cambridge, MA, USA, 2011; pp. 233–249.
40. Anderson, S.L.; Anderson, M. *Towards a principle-based healthcare agent, In Machine Medical Ethics*; van Rysewyk, S.P., Pontier, M., Eds.; Springer: Berlin/Heidelberg, Germany, 2015; pp. 67–78.
41. Coeckelbergh, M. Artificial agents, good care, and modernity. *Theor. Med. Bioeth.* **2015**, *36*, 265–277.
42. Tonkens, R. Ethics of robotic assisted dying. In *Machine Medical Ethics*; van Rysewyk, S.P., Pontier, M., Eds.; Springer: Berlin/Heidelberg, Germany, 2015; pp. 207–232.
43. van Rysewyk, S.P.; Pontier, M. A hybrid bottom-up and top-down approach to machine medical ethics: Theory and data. In *Machine Medical Ethics*; Van Rysewyk, S.P., Pontier, M., Eds.; Springer: Berlin/Heidelberg, Germany, 2015; pp. 93–110.
44. Whitby, B. Automating medicine the ethical way. In *Machine Medical Ethics*; van Rysewyk, S.P., Pontier, M., Eds.; Springer: Berlin/Heidelberg, Germany, 2015; p. 233.
45. Moor, J.H. The nature, importance, and difficulty of machine ethics. *Res. Gate* **2006**, *21*, 18–21.
46. Robot ethics: The ethical and social implications of robotics. In *Intelligent Robotics and Autonomous Agents*; Lin, P., Abney, K.; Bekey, G.A. (Eds.) MIT Press: Cambridge, MA, USA, 2014.
47. Wallach, W.; Allen, C. *Moral Machines: Teaching Robots Right from Wrong*; Oxford University Press: Oxford, UK, 2010.
48. Anderson, M.; Anderson, S.L. *Machine Ethics*; Cambridge University Press: Cambridge, MA, USA, 2011.
49. Gunkel, D.J.; Bryson, J. The machine as moral agent and patient. *Philos. Technol.* **2014**, *27*, 5–142.
50. Anderson, S.L. Machine metaethics. In *Machine Ethics*; Anderson, M., Anderson, S.L., Eds.; Cambridge University Press: Cambridge, MA, USA, 2011; pp. 21–27.
51. Finocchiaro, G. Protection of privacy and cyber risk in healthcare. *Pharm. Policy Law.* **2018**, *19*, 121–123.
52. Directive 2001/95/EC of the European Parliament and of the Council of 3 December 2001 on General Product Safety 2001. Available online: https://eur-lex.europa.eu/legal-content/EN/TXT/?uri=celex%3A52003PC0048 (accessed on 25 November 2021).
53. Regulation (EU) 2017/745 of the European Parliament and of the Council of 5 April 2017 on Medical Devices, amending Directive 2001/83/EC, Regulation (EC) No 178/2002 and Regulation (EC) No 1223/2009 and Repealing Council Directives 90/385/EEC and 93/42/EEC.2017. Available online: https://eur-lex.europa.eu/legal-content/EN/TXT/HTML/?uri=CELEX:32017R0745&from=IT (accessed on 25 November 2021).
54. NIS Directive (The Directive on Security of Network and Information Systems). Available online: https://www.itgovernance.eu/fi-fi/nis-directive-fi (accessed on 25 November 2021).
55. Complete Guide to GDPR Compliance. Available online: https://gdpr.eu/ (accessed on 25 November 2021).
56. Shaping Europe's Digital Future. Available online: https://digital-strategy.ec.europa.eu/en/policies/cybersecurity-act (accessed on 25 November 2021).
57. Fraiche, A.M.; Matlock, D.D.; Gabriel, W.; Rapley, F.A.; Kramer, D.B. Patient and provider perspectives on remote monitoring of pacemakers and implantable cardioverter-defibrillators. *Am. J. Cardiol.* **2021**, *149*, 42–46. [CrossRef]
58. Tomaiko, E.; Zawaneh, M.S. Cybersecurity threats to cardiac implantable devices:room for improvement. *Curr. Opin. Cardiol.* **2021**, *36*, 1–4. [CrossRef]
59. Saxon, L.A.; Varma, N.; Epstein, L.M.; Ganz, L.I.; Epstein, A.E. Rates of adoption and outcomes after firmware updates for food and drug administration cybersecurity safety advisories. *Circ. Arrhythm. Electrophysiol.* **2020**, *13*, e008364. [CrossRef]
60. Burnside, M.; Crocket, H.; Mayo, M.; Pickering, J.; Tappe, A.; de Bock, M. Do-it-yourself automated insulin delivery: A leading example of the democratization of medicine. *J. Diabetes Sci. Technol.* **2020**, *14*, 878–882. [CrossRef]

61. Woldaregay, A.Z.; Årsand, E.; Walderhaug, S.; Albers, D.; Mamykina, L.; Botsis, T.; Hartvigsen, G. Data-driven modeling and prediction of blood glucose dynamics:Machine learning applications in type 1 diabetes. *Artif. Intell. Med.* **2019**, *98*, 109–134. [CrossRef]
62. DeBoer, M.D.; Breton, M.D.; Wakeman, C.; Schertz, E.M.; Emory, E.G.; Robic, J.L.; Kollar, L.L.; Kovatchev, B.P.; Cherñavvsky, D.R. Performance of an artificial pancreas system for young children with type 1 diabetes. *Diabetes Technol. Ther.* **2017**, *19*, 293–298. [CrossRef]
63. Gaikwad, N.B.; Ugale, H.; Keskar, A.; Shivaprakash, N.C. The internet of battlefield things (IoBT) based enemy localization using soldiers location and gunshot direction. *IEEE Internet Things J.* **2020**, *7*, 11725–11734.
64. Tehranipoor, M.; Koushanfar, F. A survey of hardware Trojan taxonomy and detection. *IEEE Des. Test Comput* **2010**, *27*, 10–25.
65. Wang, X.; Mal-Sarkar, T.; Krishna, A.; Narasimhan, S.; Bhunia, S. Software exploitable hardware Trojans in embedded processor. In *2012 IEEE International Symposium on Defect and Fault Tolerance in VLSI and Nanotechnology Systems (DFT)*; IEEE: Piscataway Township, NJ, USA, 2012; pp. 55–58.
66. Elmiligi, H.; Gebali, F.; El-Kharashi, M.W. Multi-dimensional analysis of embedded systems security. *Microprocess. Microsyst.* **2016**, *41*, 29–36.
67. Clark, G.W.; Doran, M.V.; Andel, T.R. Cybersecurity issues in robotics. In *2017 IEEE Conference on Cognitive and Computational Aspects of Situation Management (CogSIMA)*; IEEE: Piscataway Township, NJ, USA, 2017; pp. 1–5.
68. Falliere, N.; Murchu, L.O.; Chien, E. W32. stuxnet dossier.White paper, Symantec Corp. *Secur. Response* **2011**, *5*, 29.
69. Fruhlinger, J. What is Wannacry Ransomware, How does It Infect, and Who Was Responsible. 2017. Available online: https://www.csoonline.com/article/3227906/what-is-wannacry-ransomware-how-does-it-infect-and-who-was-responsible.html (accessed on 25 November 2021).
70. Bellovin, S.M.; Merritt, M. Encrypted key exchange: Password based protocols secure against dictionary attacks. In *1992 IEEE Computer Society Symposium on Research in Security and Privacy*; IEEE: Piscataway Township, NJ, USA, 1992; pp. 72–84.
71. Kc, G.S.; Keromytis, A.D.; Prevelakis, V. Countering code injection attacks with instruction-set randomization. In Proceedings of the 10th ACM Conference on Computer and Communications Security, Washington, DC, USA, 27–30 October 2003; pp. 272–280.
72. Miller, J.; Williams, A.B.; Perouli, D. A case study on the cybersecurity of social robots. In Proceedings of the Companion of the 2018 ACM/IEEE International Conference on Human–Robot Interaction, Chicago, IL, USA, 5–8 March 2018; pp. 195–196.
73. Shahbaznezhad, H.; Kolini, F.; Rashidirad, M. Employees' behavior in phishing attacks: What individual, organizational, and technological factors matter? *J. Comput. Inf. Syst.* **2020**, *61*, 1–12.
74. Alabdan, R. Phishing attacks survey: Types, vectors, and technical approaches. *Future Internet* **2020**, *12*, 168.
75. Mo, Y.; Garone, E.; Casavola, A.; Sinopoli, B. False data injection attacks against state estimation in wireless sensor networks. In *2010 49th IEEE Conference on Decision and Control (CDC)*; IEEE: Piscataway Township, NJ, USA, 2010; pp. 5967–5972.
76. Senie, D.; Ferguson, P. Network ingress filtering: Defeating denial of service attacks which employ IP source address spoofing. *Network* 1998.
77. Navas, R.E.; Le Bouder, H.; Cuppens, N.; Cuppens, F.; Papadopoulos, G.Z. Do not trust your neighbors! A small IoT platform illustrating a man-in-the-middle attack. In Proceedings of the International Conference on Ad-Hoc Networks and Wireless, St. Malo, France, 5–7 September 2018; Springer: Berlin/Heidelberg, Germany, 2018; pp. 120–125.
78. Evidence-Based Medicine Guidelines. Available online: https://www.ebm-guidelines.com/dtk/ebmg/home (accessed on 25 November 2021).
79. Luce, B.R.; Drummond, M.; Jönsson, B.; Neumann, P.J.; Schwartz, J.S.; Siebert, U.; Sullivan, S.D. EBM, HTA, and CER: Clearing the confusion. *Milbank Q.* **2010**, *88*, 256–276. [CrossRef]
80. Office of Technology Assessment. 1978. Assessing the Efficacy and Safety of Medical Technologies. September. NTIS order #PB-286929. Available online: http://www.fas.org/ota/reports/7805.pdf (accessed on 25 November 2009).
81. INAHTA (International Network of Agencies for Health Technology Assessment). HTA Resources. 2009. Available online: http://www.inahta.org/HTA/ (accessed on 25 November 2009).
82. Candiani, G.; Colombo, C.; Daghini, R.; Magrini, N. Come Organizzare una Conferenza di Consenso. Manuale Metodologico, Roma, ISS-SNLG. 2009. Available online: https://www.psy.it/wp-content/uploads/2018/02/Manuale-Metodologico-Consensus.pdf (accessed on 25 November 2021).
83. Arcelloni, M.C.; Milani, C. Consensus Conference: Uno Strumento per la Pratica Clinica Riferimenti Storico-Metodologici e Stato Dell'arte dei Lavori Italiani sul Disturbo Primario del Linguaggio e sui Disturbi Specifici dell'Apprendimento. Available online: https://rivistedigitali.erickson.it/il-tnpee/archivio/vol-1-n-1/riferimenti-storico-metodologici-e-stato-dellarte-dei-lavori-italiani-sul-disturbo-primario-del-linguaggio-e-sui-disturbi-specifici-dellapprendimento/ (accessed on 25 November 2021).
84. McGlynn, E.A.; Kosecoff, J.; Brook, R.H. Format and conduct of consensus development conferences. Multi-nation comparison. *Int. J. Technol. Assess Health Care* **1990**, *6*, 450–469. [CrossRef]

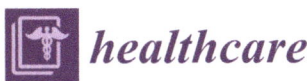

Comment

Comment on Anwer et al. Rehabilitation of Upper Limb Motor Impairment in Stroke: A Narrative Review on the Prevalence, Risk Factors, and Economic Statistics of Stroke and State of the Art Therapies. *Healthcare* 2022, *10*, 190

Giovanni Morone [1] and Daniele Giansanti [2,*]

1. Department of Life, Health and Environmental Sciences, University of L'Aquila, 67100 L'Aquila, Italy; giovanni.morone@univaq.it
2. Centre Tisp, The Italian National Institute of Health, 00161 Rome, Italy
* Correspondence: daniele.giansanti@iss.it; Tel.: +39-06-49902701

We are writing to you as the corresponding author of the interesting review study entitled "Rehabilitation of Upper Limb Motor Impairment in Stroke: A Narrative Review on the Prevalence, Risk Factors, and Economic Statistics of Stroke and State of the Art Therapies" [1].

We found that this work is particularly stimulating and provides a great added value to the field.

Specifically, we believe that this review has the great merit of focusing on both key aspects of the integration of upper limb rehabilitation in the *health domain* and aspects relating to technological innovation, including, in addition to purely clinical aspects, economic aspects and risk factors.

In the Special Issue (SI) [2,3] "*Rehabilitation and Robotics: Are They Working Well Together?*" we addressed these issues with reference to the use of robotic technologies. In particular, we focused on clinical studies on the use of robotic technologies in the rehabilitation field, ranging from the field of disabling pathologies of neurological origin to the field of injuries, also including the support of the elderly (in particular, frail persons) or of people with communication disabilities. It must be borne in mind that, in the robotics sector, despite major developments there is no uniformity or standardization of use. Robotics is often used on a very limited basis to pilot and/or research projects. The purpose of the Special Issue was to take stock of the issues that hinder the integration of robotics in clinical practice and on useful initiatives in this direction. We consider your study to be very important for having faced, along with many other themes, the theme of the robotics. Your analytical study reviewed different technologies used for therapies such as functional electric stimulation, noninvasive brain stimulation including transcranial direct current stimulation, transcranial magnetic stimulation, invasive epidural cortical stimulation, virtual reality rehabilitation, robot-assisted training, and telerehabilitation. These technologies can be used alone or even in synergy. As an example, robotics is currently also used in telerehabilitation.

The review highlighted, in line with the SI [2,3], both the potential of robotics in perspective and its limits.

Among potential applications, it was highlighted how:

- Pilot studies [4] have shown promisingly positive results of robot-assisted rehabilitation for recovery and plasticity following a stroke.
- Assistive technologies (robotic prosthetic limbs and devices) are useful and promising for supporting the human body's lost function [5].

The limits and perplexities of the effectiveness of the use of robotics in comparison with other traditional therapies were also highlighted. Some included studies reported that such comparisons in some applications:

- Were positive but not satisfactory [6].
- Did not reveal a significant improvement of upper limb functionalities [7–11].

Robotics as a single technology or integrated with other different biomedical technologies [1], ranging from functional electric stimulation to telerehabilitation, represents an important perspective of research in this field for scholars.

In this same field, very recent studies [12–14] have addressed the potential of technologies based on artificial intelligence (AI) in neurological rehabilitation applications based on robotics. AI looks promising for both face-to-face rehabilitation [12,13] and remote activities [14].

The study by Yang et al. [12] described how the rapid development of intelligent computing has attracted the attention of researchers of robotic neurorehabilitation with computational intelligence, reporting that Artificial Intelligence affected both the mechanical structures and the control methods in rehabilitation robotics.

The study by Nizamiz et al. [13] pointed out how novel, wearable robotic devices are being tailored to specific patient populations, such as those with traumatic brain injury, stroke, and amputation, and how AI could facilitate the developments in robot-assisted rehabilitation in motor learning and in generating movement repetitions by decoding the brain activity of patients during therapy.

The study by Lambercy et al. [14] faced the perspective of robot-assisted therapy in a minimally supervised and decentralized manner, using rehabilitation devices that are portable, scalable, and equipped with clinical intelligence, remote monitoring, and coaching capabilities.

Considering the research you have undertaken, we would like to hear your opinion about that, and, in particular, if you think that among current and future developments, AI will play an important role in this sector in an autonomous contribution and/or in support of the technologies mentioned in your review study.

We would strongly appreciate an opinion on this as a reply in the SI.

Funding: This research received no external funding.

Institutional Review Board Statement: Not applicable.

Informed Consent Statement: Not applicable.

Data Availability Statement: Not applicable.

Conflicts of Interest: The authors declare no conflict of interest.

References

1. Anwer, S.; Waris, A.; Gilani, S.O.; Iqbal, J.; Shaikh, N.; Pujari, A.N.; Niazi, I.K. Rehabilitation of Upper Limb Motor Impairment in Stroke: A Narrative Review on the Prevalence, Risk Factors, and Economic Statistics of Stroke and State of the Art Therapies. *Healthcare* **2022**, *10*, 190. [CrossRef]
2. Available online: https://www.mdpi.com/journal/healthcare/special_issues/Robotic_Rehabilitation (accessed on 17 April 2022).
3. Giansanti, D. The Rehabilitation and the Robotics: Are They Going Together Well? *Healthcare* **2021**, *9*, 26. [CrossRef] [PubMed]
4. Blank, A.A.; French, J.A.; Pehlivan, A.U.; O'Malley, M.K. Current trends in robot-assisted upper-limb stroke rehabilitation: Promoting patient engagement in therapy. *Curr. Phys. Med. Rehabil. Rep.* **2014**, *2*, 184–195. [CrossRef] [PubMed]
5. McFarland, D.J.; Wolpaw, J.R. Brain-computer interface operation of robotic and prosthetic devices. *Computer* **2008**, *41*, 52–56. [CrossRef]
6. Masiero, S.; Poli, P.; Rosati, G.; Zanotto, D.; Iosa, M.; Paolucci, S.; Morone, G. The value of robotic systems in stroke rehabilitation. *Expert Rev. Med. Devices* **2014**, *11*, 187–198. [CrossRef] [PubMed]
7. Veerbeek, J.M.; Langbroek-Amersfoort, A.C.; VanWegen, E.E.; Meskers, C.G.; Kwakkel, G. Effects of robot-assisted therapy for the upper limb after stroke: A systematic review and meta-analysis. *Neurorehabil. Neural Repair* **2017**, *31*, 107–121. [CrossRef] [PubMed]
8. Morone, G.; Paolucci, S.; Cherubini, A.; De Angelis, D.; Venturiero, V.; Coiro, P.; Iosa, M. Robot-assisted gait training for stroke patients: Current state of the art and perspectives of robotics. *Neuropsychiatric Dis. Treat.* **2017**, *13*, 1303. [CrossRef] [PubMed]

9. Mehrholz, J.; Pohl, M.; Platz, T.; Kugler, J.; Elsner, B. Electromechanical and robot-assisted arm training for improving activities of daily living, arm function, and arm muscle strength after stroke. *Cochrane Database Syst. Rev.* **2018**, *9*, CD006876. [CrossRef] [PubMed]
10. Rodgers, H.; Bosomworth, H.; Krebs, H.I.; van Wijck, F.; Howel, D.; Wilson, N.; Shaw, L. Robot assisted training for the upper limb after stroke (RATULS): A multicentre randomised controlled trial. *Lancet* **2019**, *394*, 51–62. [CrossRef]
11. Fasoli, S.E.; Adans-Dester, C.P. A paradigm shift: Rehabilitation robotics, cognitive skills training, and function after stroke. *Front. Neurol.* **2019**, *10*, 1088. [CrossRef] [PubMed]
12. Yang, J.; Zhao, Z.; Du, C.; Wang, W.; Peng, Q.; Qiu, J.; Wang, G. The realization of robotic neurorehabilitation in future prospects analysis. *Expert Rev. Med. Devices* **2020**, *17*, 1311–1322. [CrossRef] [PubMed]
13. Nizamis, K.; Athanasiou, A.; Almpani, S.; Dimitrousis, C.; Astaras, A. Converging Robotic Technologies in Targeted Neural Rehabilitation: A Review of Emerging Solutions and Challenges. *Sensors* **2021**, *21*, 2084. [CrossRef] [PubMed]
14. Lambercy, O.; Lehner, R.; Chua, K.; Wee, S.K.; Rajeswaran, D.K.; Kuah, C.W.K.; Ang, W.T.; Liang, P.; Campolo, D.; Hussain, A.; et al. Neurorehabilitation From a Distance: Can Intelligent Technology Support Decentralized Access to Quality Therapy? *Front. Robot* **2021**, *8*, 612415. [CrossRef] [PubMed]

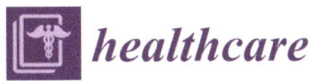

Reply

Reply to Morone, G.; Giansanti, D. Comment on "Anwer et al. Rehabilitation of Upper Limb Motor Impairment in Stroke: A Narrative Review on the Prevalence, Risk Factors, and Economic Statistics of Stroke and State of the Art Therapies. *Healthcare* 2022, 10, 190"

Saba Anwer [1], Asim Waris [1], Syed Omer Gilani [1], Javaid Iqbal [1], Nusratnaaz Shaikh [2], Amit N. Pujari [3,4] and Imran Khan Niazi [2,5,6,*]

1. School of Mechanical & Manufacturing Engineering, National University of Sciences and Technology (NUST), Islamabad 45200, Pakistan; sanwer.bmes19smme@student.nust.edu.pk (S.A.); asim.waris@smme.nust.edu.pk (A.W.); omer@smme.nust.edu.pk (S.O.G.); j.iqbal@ceme.nust.edu.pk (J.I.)
2. Faculty of Health & Environmental Sciences, Health & Rehabilitation Research Institute, AUT University, Auckland 0627, New Zealand; nusrat.shaikh@aut.ac.nz
3. School of Physics, Engineering and Computer Science, University of Hertfordshire, Hatfield AL10 9AB, UK; amit.pujari@ieee.org
4. School of Engineering, University of Aberdeen, Aberdeen AB24 3FX, UK
5. Center of Chiropractic Research, New Zealand College of Chiropractic, Auckland 1060, New Zealand
6. Center for Sensory-Motor Interaction, Department of Health Science & Technology, Aalborg University, 9000 Alborg, Denmark
* Correspondence: imran.niazi@nzchiro.co.nz

Thank you so much for your kind remarks. We really appreciate your detailed analysis [1] of this review study [2]. The use of robotics based on the concept of artificial intelligence in the field of rehabilitation is really an interesting subject, and it will be a pleasure for us to give an opinion on this issue.

Firstly, it is very important to understand that, with the increasing rate of stroke-related disability, it will be difficult to provide stroke survivors with post-stroke care (PSC) services because of their unbearable economic consequences, which raises the need to minimize the role of physical therapists and move towards adopting self-rehabilitative home-based therapies to facilitate healthcare for those living in remote areas.

Secondly, the rehabilitation field is shifting from conventional approaches to new and technologically advanced therapeutic strategies in which virtual reality, telerehabilitation, robotics, and invasive and non-invasive stimulations are top of the list.

For the use of artificial intelligence to fabricate modern medical equipment such as prosthetic limbs, robotic machinery is inevitable. Such systems are strongly bound with the commitment to making rehabilitation systems more comfortable, with a significantly increased degree of freedom for stroke patients or victims of limb amputations.

As An example, I will mention a commercially available system of Saebo-VR (https://www.saebo.com/virtual-reality/) (accessed on 28 March 2022) which is an interactive, multisensory computer-based simulation environment providing the patients with an opportunity to perform different activities in the real world. Saebo also provides a cutting-edge Saeb Glove (https://uk.saebo.com/shop/saeboglove/) (accessed on 28 March 2022) which helps its users suffering from different orthopedic and neurological injuries to incorporate with their motor therapy for assistance at home. This proprietary tension system assists patients to perform finger extension following a grasp action. This fully functional, commercially available setup is a bewildering example of AI-based robot-assisted system for patients with motor disabilities.

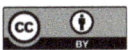

Moreover, systems such as Microsoft Kinect play significant roles in physiotherapy and rehabilitation of stroke patients. Microsoft Kinect device (https://www.physio-pedia.com/The_emerging_role_of_Microsoft_Kinect_in_physiotherapy_rehabilitation_for_stroke_patients) (accessed on 28 March 2022) offers exciting and innovative ways of rehabilitation that make the treatment, and thus the subsequent adherence and motivation, more interactive and enjoyable. Microsoft Kinect allows stroke survivors suffering from motor disabilities to interact with an environment where they can perform different movement combinations without any need for a controller or attached device.

This review article provides an overview of, and deep insights into, modern alternative rehabilitation technologies. Moreover, the review article focuses on the importance of stroke rehabilitation while narratively explaining the socio-economic burden of this disease and related risk factors. Considering the increasing popularity and evidence of the benefits of technology-aided rehabilitation approaches, some commonly used stroke therapies to regain muscle activity are discussed. The reader can refer to the cited articles for more information.

Despite all presented discussions, we cannot deny the fact that the future is strongly associated with excess use of artificial intelligence in the field of rehabilitation—whether it is telerehabilitation, virtual reality, robot-assisted therapies, or participatory involvement of multiple techniques. Hopefully, I have answered the question. For more details, please refer to the cited article [2–5].

Author Contributions: S.A. and A.W. presented the concept and design of the paper. S.O.G., J.I., I.K.N. and N.S. helped in the authentic data collection from different research databases. A.W., S.A. and A.N.P. drafted the manuscript. All the authors thoroughly studied and approved the final manuscript. All authors have read and agreed to the published version of the manuscript.

Funding: This research received no external funding.

Institutional Review Board Statement: Not applicable.

Informed Consent Statement: Not applicable.

Data Availability Statement: Data presented in the paper is extracted from published work. The authors of the current study do not have the raw data.

Conflicts of Interest: Authors declare no conflict of interest.

References

1. Morone, G.; Giansanti, D. Comment on Anwer et al. Rehabilitation of Upper Limb Motor Impairment in Stroke: A Narrative Review on the Prevalence, Risk Factors, and Economic Statistics of Stroke and State of the Art Therapies. *Healthcare* 2022, *10*, 190. *Healthcare* **2022**, *10*, 846. [CrossRef]
2. Anwer, S.; Waris, A.; Gilani, S.O.; Iqbal, J.; Shaikh, N.; Pujari, A.N.; Niazi, I.K. Rehabilitation of Upper Limb Motor Impairment in Stroke: A Narrative Review on the Prevalence, Risk Factors, and Economic Statistics of Stroke and State of the Art Therapies. *Healthcare* **2022**, *10*, 190. [CrossRef] [PubMed]
3. Masiero, S.; Poli, P.; Rosati, G.; Zanotto, D.; Iosa, M.; Paolucci, S.; Morone, G. The value of robotic systems in stroke rehabilitation. *Expert Rev. Med. Devices* **2014**, *11*, 187–198. [CrossRef] [PubMed]
4. Veerbeek, J.M.; Langbroek-Amersfoort, A.C.; VanWegen, E.E.; Meskers, C.G.; Kwakkel, G. Effects of robot-assisted therapy for the upper limb after stroke: A systematic review and meta-analysis. *Neurorehabil. Neural Repair.* **2017**, *31*, 107–121. [CrossRef] [PubMed]
5. Vélez-Guerrero, M.A.; Callejas-Cuervo, M.; Mazzoleni, S. Artificial intelligence-based wearable robotic exoskeletons for upper limb rehabilitation: A review. *Sensors* **2021**, *21*, 2146. [CrossRef] [PubMed]

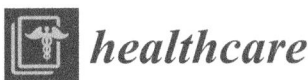

Article

Ethics and Automated Systems in the Health Domain: Design and Submission of a Survey on Rehabilitation and Assistance Robotics to Collect Insiders' Opinions and Perception

Giovanni Morone [1], Antonia Pirrera [2], Paola Meli [2] and Daniele Giansanti [2,*]

[1] Dipartimento di Medicina Clinica, Sanità Pubblica, Scienze della Vita e dell'Ambiente, Università degli Studi dell'Aquila, 67100 L'Aquila, Italy; giovanni.morone@univaq.it

[2] Centro TISP, Istituto Superiore di Sanità, 00161 Roma, Italy; antonia.pirrera@iss.it (A.P.); paola.meli@iss.it (P.M.)

* Correspondence: daniele.giansanti@iss.it

Abstract: Background: The problem of the relationship between ethics and robotics is very broad, has important implications, and has two large areas of impact: the first is conduct in research, development, and use in general. The second is the implication of the programming of machine ethics. Purpose: Develop and administer a survey of professionals in the health domain collection of their positions on ethics in rehabilitation and assistance robotics. Methods: An electronic survey was designed using Microsoft Forms and submitted to 155 professionals in the health domain (age between 23 and 64 years; 78 males, mean age 43.7, minimum age 24, maximum age 64; 77 females, mean age 44.3, minimum age 23, maximum age 64) using social media. Results and discussion: The outcome returned: (a) the position on ethics training during university studies and in the world of work, (b) the organizational aspects hindered by ethics and those to be perfected in relation to ethics, (c) issues of ethical concern, (d) structured feedback on the usefulness of the methodology along with considerations of open text. Conclusions: An electronic survey methodology has allowed the structured collection of information on positions towards ethics in this sector. Encouraging feedback from the participants suggests the continuation of the study is beneficial. A continuation is expected, expanding the audience of professionals involved and perfecting the survey with the support of scientific companies.

Keywords: ethics; robotics; social robot; rehabilitation

Citation: Morone, G.; Pirrera, A.; Meli, P.; Giansanti, D. Ethics and Automated Systems in the Health Domain: Design and Submission of a Survey on Rehabilitation and Assistance Robotics to Collect Insiders' Opinions and Perception. *Healthcare* **2022**, *10*, 778. https://doi.org/10.3390/healthcare10050778

Academic Editor: Joaquim Carreras

Received: 11 March 2022
Accepted: 16 April 2022
Published: 22 April 2022

Publisher's Note: MDPI stays neutral with regard to jurisdictional claims in published maps and institutional affiliations.

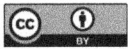

Copyright: © 2022 by the authors. Licensee MDPI, Basel, Switzerland. This article is an open access article distributed under the terms and conditions of the Creative Commons Attribution (CC BY) license (https://creativecommons.org/licenses/by/4.0/).

1. Introduction

1.1. Robotics in Rehabilitation and Assistance

The Policy Department for Economic, Scientific and Quality of Life Policies of the European Parliament identified the most interesting applications of the care robots (CR)s [1]. The international body identified the following sectors:

1. Robotic surgery
2. Care and socially assistive robots
3. Rehabilitation systems
4. Training for health and care workers.

These sector are varied. Numbers two and three are both sectors connected to rehabilitation and assistance. Rehabilitation robotics are utilized in three areas [2]: (a) balance, (b) the lower limbs, and (c) the upper limbs. Two different technological solutions are used, based on exoskeleton technology and end-effector technology, with different implications in application [3]. Social robots are used in several multifaceted fields of the health domain for assistance and rehabilitation, including psychological, physical, and neurological rehabilitation [4].

1.2. Ethics and the Introduction of the Automated Systems in the Health Domain

The introduction of decision-making, therapeutic, and rehabilitation approaches, based on automatic systems, is radically changing the perspective of care in the health domain, raising important questions from an ethical point of view. As highlighted in [5], the use of automated systems in biomedical and clinical settings can disrupt the traditional doctor–patient relationship, which is based on the trust and transparency of medical advice and therapeutic decisions. An important criticism in [5] is that this approach, in which clinical decisions are no longer made solely by the physician, but to a significant extent by a machine using algorithms, decisions become non-transparent. They proposed a more ethical approach in which the decisions of these automatic systems are transparent, even to insiders. On the other hand, digital health is pushing towards an increasingly marked integration in the health domain, and access to healthcare records is more possible and easier than ever. All of this allows for the integration of automated systems and has the potential to transform medicine. To cite some examples: (a) Identifying previously unknown interventions that reduce the risk of adverse outcomes [6,7]. (b) Integration into medical decision workflows, from cellular and histological diagnostics [8] to functional and diagnostic imaging of organs [9], where scholars have highlighted how ethics is one of the most important challenges [10]. (c) Working in direct contact with patients through robots and other solutions based on artificial intelligence, where the implications, precisely for this reason, are broad and multifaceted [11]. Considering this, a conscious approach to ethics is now mandatory.

1.3. Ethics and Rehabilitation and Assistance Robotics

The issues of the ethics of automatic systems in the health domain are generally applicable to rehabilitation and assistance robotics. Rehabilitation and assistance robotics partially share ethical issues with automated systems; however, ethical issues in the latter field have also some peculiarities, such as direct work with patients [11]. The problem of the relationship between ethics and robotics is very broad and has important implications, ranging from integration of consent to cybersecurity [12].

Ethics in the field of rehabilitation and assistance robotics has two large areas of impact to many issues, which are shared with automatic systems in general. The first large dimension is research conduct, development, and use in general [13,14]. This concerns both social robots and robots in used in rehabilitation [15,16]. The second large dimension concerns only social robots and is the design of machine ethics [17].

Regarding the first dimension, Stahl and Coeckelbergh [13] identified, as a first important topic, the technological impact to daily life and the health domain. The implications of replacing humans with machines in the health domain must be addressed [18–25]. Therefore, the following issues are of particular importance:

- the implications to work of those in contact with the patient;
- consequently, the quality of care in relation to what has been defined as a risk of dehumanization or even cold care.

When focusing on the replacement, of humans it is necessary to consider:

- the implications of the decision-making autonomy of the decision-making robot (e.g., margins and impact);
- the chain of responsibility for the decision-making robot;
- the risk of deception, such as the risk of creating false friendships with social robots;
- the trust in placing a patient (for example a frail person) in the hands of a robot.

Then there is a second important topic, connected with the cybersecurity applied to the mechatronic. The following issues are important:

- privacy and data protection;
- safety and avoidance of harm.

Gordon highlighted a second large dimension [17], which addresses the problems of ethics when implementing ethical rules in a moral robot. All this is important to broad and interdisciplinary sectors, such as artificial intelligence. The criticality of this sector is given by the fact that anyone who programs ethics in a computer must have specific training on ethics [26–29].

Etemad-Sajadi et al. [30] also categorized (after a review of the state of the art) six specific strategic items of concern related to ethics in this sector, which must be taken into consideration in studies on the integration of consent: social cues [21,22,28,29], trust and safety [13,30], autonomy [13,30,31], replacement [30,32–34], responsibility [13,30,34], and privacy and data protection [13,30,35].

Robotics in this sector have also developed a strong integration with virtual reality [3] and is moving towards an important integration with artificial intelligence [36]. When we focus on ethics, we must even consider pursuits such as these.

Furthermore, we must not forget an emerging ethical issue in automatic systems in general which is also applicable here: the implication of equity [37]. Health systems rely on commercial prediction algorithms to identify and help patients with complex health needs. In [37], it was shown that a widely used algorithm in automated systems, affecting millions of patients, exhibited significant racial bias. This must be particularly considered and avoided even in robotics, which has already been used in the health domain as a niche rehabilitation and assistance system.

1.4. Hypothesis of the Study

Ethics is assuming an essential and important role in the introduction of rehabilitation and assistance robotics in the health domain. It is therefore crucial to consider the ethics in studies on the integration of consensus.

Professionals who are involved in patient interaction will increasingly play a key role in interacting with robotics in a wide range of activities, ranging from the execution of robotics-based protocols to application programming in robots. The ethics of the integration of rehabilitation and assistance robotics is passed through the opinions and consent of these professionals.

We hypothesized that it was possible to focus on these figures and to remotely administer, through the mobile technology, an electronic survey to collect demographic data and to collect information on professionals' training and their relationships with ethics.

1.5. Objectives of the Study

- Develop and administer a remote electronic survey that would allow: (a) the collection of demographic data and (b) the collection of data on the training on ethics and the self-perception of the impact of the ethics, concerns, and suggestions.
- To collect feedback on the investigation and opinions on this topic.

2. Methods

2.1. Participants and Procedure

2.1.1. The Selected Tool and the Adequacy of Regulations

This questionnaire project was previously carefully discussed with experts on data protection. It complies to regulations (national and international) of the European GDPR 679/2016 and the Italian Decree 101/2018. The questionnaire was anonymous, and the topic did not concern clinical trials on humans or animals. Furthermore, it did not involve participants with pathologies. In consideration of this, after a pre-check, the approval of an ethics committee was not deemed necessary (which would have required a long time, incompatible with this study). However, to improve the privacy aspects, we did not proceed via e-mail and to avoid requesting the municipality of residence (in small municipalities, this it could lead to identification). In this study, the software Microsoft Forms was chosen. Our company has this tool centrally installed. Users have this tool, among other applications, on the Microsoft 365 App Business Premium suite (the maximum limit of participants/submission is 50,000). All users, internal and external, can access through their own domain account guaranteed by corporate cybersecurity standards (which are forced to comply with international regulations) to develop surveys by Forms. The developed products, shared with external subjects, are supported in each phase both by the system security tools/system policy and network security, managed by the company firewall, which can also perform specific checks on the IPs (registering, for example, duplicate access for further data processing). The data acquired through a survey developed by means of Microsoft Forms, are protected by corporate security systems. In fact, they are a register for legal purposes in case of the presence of sensitive data (for which the creator of the survey is responsible) and are protected by corporate cyber security systems, guaranteeing (at least from the system point of view) the inviolability of the data and the maintenance, according to article five of the GDPR 679/2016, for a period of time not exceeding the achievement of the purposes for which they are processed. Microsoft Forms is the tool recommended by the company's Data Protection Office. A choice different than Forms would have required a specific report and cybersecurity study; therefore, the authorization to use it would not have been guaranteed. The use of both an internal recommended tool (respecting the cybersecurity) and the choice to submit the survey anonymously (without requiring sensitive data) simplified the process of launch, that, after a preliminary check, did not need specific authorizations.

2.1.2. Main Characteristics of the Chosen Tool

The chosen electronic survey (Microsoft Forms), based on the above considerations, allows submission via an internet link accessible in a secure manner, reported above by means of an https link. This tool allows sending via multimedia systems, chats, emails, webs, social networks, in a simple way, and data collection automatically. It avoids all laborious paper submission activities as well as laborious data collection, not free from errors, due to transcription from paper to an electronic database for processing.

Once sent by the administrator, the electronic survey is opened by the receiver, filled in, and by means of a simple sending confirmation, allows the data to be uploaded in real time into a database. At any time, and in particular at the fixed and scheduled deadline for sending replies, data are accessible both in the form of post-processing reports and in Microsoft Excel for other statistical post-processing analyses.

An example of this flow is shown in Figure 1, where the submission is illustrated using one of the possible tools (WhatsApp).

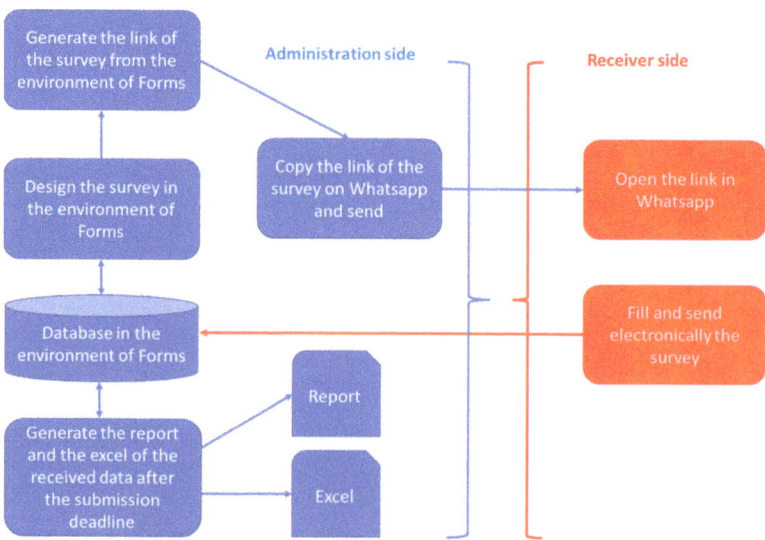

Figure 1. An example of the submission flow based on a possible applicable tool (WhatsApp).

A subtitle can also be inserted on each question that guides the compiler giving greater certainty and security on what to insert. In [38,39], where there are links and pdf printouts of the survey (described in the following), you can see, for example: (a) A subtitle of the heading, before the questions of the survey reports, "The survey is dedicated to the healthcare professionals. It is anonymous. The submitted data are protected by cybersecurity.-PLEASE help those who are not technology experts to fill in the questionnaire-" giving information and clarifications (also on security aspects). (b) In the first question, a subtitle gives clarifications and information on the security to the participants. (c) A subtitle helps the participants in the second question.

2.1.3. The Tool: Structure

The tool included four sections: (a) A section dedicated to the information of the participants, asking for consent to the survey, information related to demographic data (sex, age), and a brief curriculum. (b) A section with graded questions and Likert scales [40] dedicated to self-perception of the training and impact of ethics in, e.g., concerns and suggestions in the workplace. (c) A section with graded and open questions asking for opinions on the methodology.

The original survey is in Italian and is closed and no longer accessible.

We have translated a version from Italian into English for editorial purposes. A link to the interactive tool is available online at [38].

The link to the pdf printout is available online at [39].

2.1.4. Submission and Participants

The only prerequisite that we set ourselves, to limit the articulations of the study, was to focus on healthcare professionals (graduates in occupational therapy, physiotherapy, orthopaedic techniques, nursing, rehabilitation, and similar courses). Based on a dedicated section, respondents were included (or excluded) according to compliance (or non-compliance) with these requirements (Figure 2).

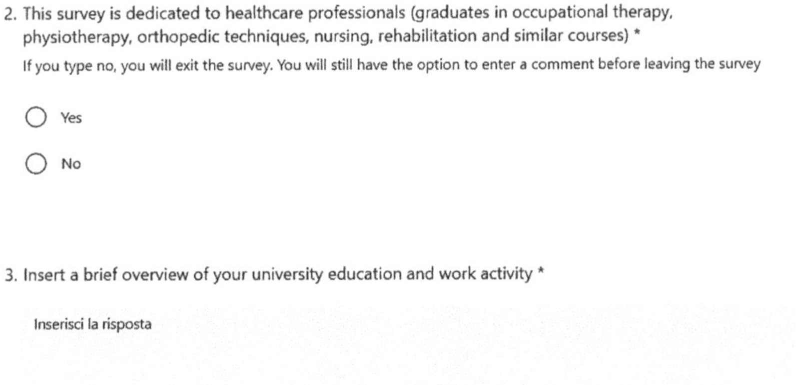

2. This survey is dedicated to healthcare professionals (graduates in occupational therapy, physiotherapy, orthopedic techniques, nursing, rehabilitation and similar courses) *

If you type no, you will exit the survey. You will still have the option to enter a comment before leaving the survey

○ Yes

○ No

3. Insert a brief overview of your university education and work activity *

Inserisci la risposta

Figure 2. The section of the questionnaire dedicated to inclusion in the study.

The electronic survey was sent on 15 October 2021. The tool remained active until 15 December 2021. The submission took place through social media, such as Facebook, LinkedIn, Twitter, Instagram, WhatsApp, association sites or scientific societies, and in general, a peer-to-peer dissemination.

We have also encouraged both the spread of the electronic survey and the support in filling out for those who are less familiar with digital technology (also strongly specifying this in the electronic survey introduction).

Table 1 shows the demographic characteristics of the participants in the study.

Table 1. Demographics characteristics.

Participants	Age and Gender
155 professionals of the health domain with specific academic training	Age between 23 and 64 years. 78 males (mean age 43.7; minimum age 24, maximum age 64) 77 females (mean age 44.3; minimum age 23, maximum age 64)

2.2. Measures

The survey considered various parameters for the collection and evaluation of information, some of which were used in this work and others will be explored further later. The following parameters were considered to be related to the submission rate: the total submissions, the total number of people who opened the survey but didn't participate, the total number of those who could not be included, and the total number of people.

In the survey there are also graded questions and open questions (for comments) to have feedback on the administration process. We established a six-level psychometric scale for the graded questions. The assignable values ranged from a minimum score = 1 to a maximum score = 6. Considering this, a theoretical average value (TMV) can be identified as:

$$TMV = \frac{1+6}{2} = 3.5 \qquad (1)$$

The value in Equation (1) is equally distant, with an absolute value of 2.5 both from the maximum assignable score = 6 and the minimum assignable score = 1.

It is therefore possible to assign a minimum score of one and a maximum of six with a theoretical mean value (TMV) of 3.5. We can refer to the TMV for comparison in the analysis of the answers. An average value of the answers below the TMV indicates a more negative than positive response. An average value above the TMV indicates a more positive than negative response. The outcome of the open questions was investigated qualitatively. The best five were selected on the basis of a ranking formed on the basis of an evaluation that took into account on impact and significance.

In the survey, there are also Likert scale questions (as for example the question 7, Figure 3A) and choice questions (Figure 3B). We established a six-level psychometric scale for the Likert scale questions as the graded questions.

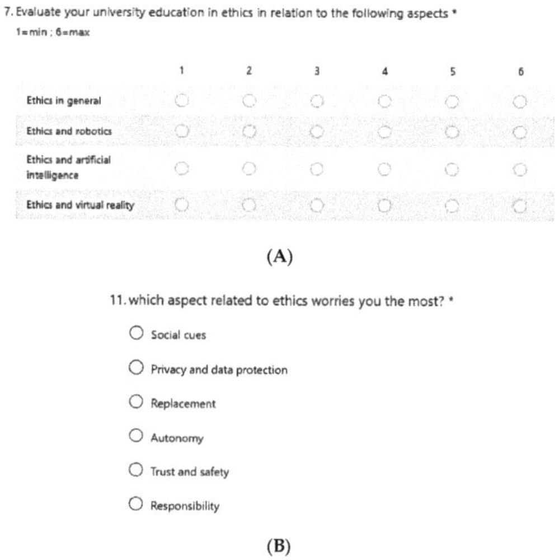

Figure 3. (**A**) Survey section (Likert's scale) dedicated to questions on academic training. (**B**) The choice question with ethical aspects of concern.

2.3. Statistics

We used the Smirnov–Kolmogorov test for testing the normality, as it is preferable for large samples such as ours. We applied the χ^2 test (with a $p < 0.01$ for the assessment of the significance) in the frequency analysis.

We applied the Student's t-test (with a $p < 0.01$ for the assessment of the significance) when investigating the difference between the parameters.

The Cohen's d effect size was estimated for the assessment of the adequacy of the sample. Furthermore, the Cronbach's α value was assessed for the psychometric sections of the electronic survey. The software SPSS version 24 was used in the study.

3. Results

The results are organized into four paragraphs. The first paragraph reports the results of the administration. The second paragraph reports a statistical analysis of significance, firstly, the statistical tests then applied to the analysis of the outcome. The third paragraph is dedicated to the central analysis of the study, i.e., the analysis of the participants' opinion/perception. The fourth paragraph reports the analysis of the participants' feedback on the method.

3.1. Submission

The electronic survey was sent on 15 October 2021. The tool remained active until October 25. A total of 91.74% of responses were obtained in the first four days. We sent 202 electronic surveys and 14 subjects did not give the consent. A total of 33 subjects could not be included because they did not pass the inclusion process reported in Figure 2. A total of 155 participants were included, as can be observed in Table 1.

3.2. Preliminary Test of Statistical Significance

Preliminarily to the analysis, we applied the selected tests to verify the normality of the data, the adequacy of the sample, and the sensitivity of individual factors.

We tested the distribution of age for the sample with the Smirnov–Kolmogorov test of normality, which is suitable for large samples such as ours. The null hypothesis was that our data followed a normal distribution. We achieved $p = 0.53$. Because $p > 0.05$, we accepted the null hypothesis. We were therefore working with a normal distribution.

The Cohen's d effect size was 0.499, indicating that the proposed sample was suitable ($N > 60$). Furthermore, the Cronbach's α value of individual factors was assessed for the graded questions and the Likert questions. It reported a value = 0.8, i.e., a good level of reliability.

3.3. The Ethics Perception on the Insiders

You can refer to [38,39] for the questions in detail.

Question no. 6, related to robotics training, reported a score of 3.61, just above the TMV. The Likert scale in question 7 (Table 2), relating to the evaluation of training on ethical aspects, reported an evaluation lower than the TMV for all modules (ethics in general, ethics and robotics, ethics and artificial intelligence, and ethics and virtual reality).

Table 2. Output from the Likert scale "Evaluate your university education in ethics in relation to the following aspects".

Question	Score
Ethics in general	3.04
Ethics and robotics	2.87
Ethics and artificial intelligence	2.93
Ethics and virtual reality	2.99

The same Likert scale applied to the current knowledge on the job (Table 3), with question number 8 [38,39], reports a better situation (above TMV for all modules), presumably thanks to the improvements in knowledge triggered in the workplace, due to a greater sensitivity determined on the issue by professional associations or scientific societies. The Student's t-test was applied to verify the significance of the difference between the same modules in the two Likert scales. The test of the four applications always reported a high significance of the difference ($p < 0.01$).

Table 3. Output from the Likert scale "Evaluate your current knowledge in ethics in relation to the following aspects".

Question	Score
Ethics in general	3.64
Ethics and robotics	3.51
Ethics and artificial intelligence	3.52
Ethics and virtual reality	3.53

In regards the two Likert questions:

9—"Regarding the organizational aspects, what would you suggest to improve in terms of training and/or in-depth study in the field of ethics in robotic rehabilitation in the neurological field?" and

10—"Regarding the organizational aspects, do you think that ethical issues can hinder ?"

We have decided to report the details of the answers together with the average values. In this manner, we can compare the frequencies of positive answers (more positive than negative: values of 4, 5, and 6) with the frequencies of the negative answers (more negative than positive: values of 1, 2, and 3).

Both Likert questions reported a higher frequency of positive responses (more positive than negative: values of 4, 5, and 6). The χ^2 applied to each of the elements of the two Likert questions always showed a high statistical significance ($p < 0.01$).

As for the Likert scale in Table 4 (question 9), all of the elements proposed showed a need for improvement in terms of training and/or in-depth study. Among the elements proposed (the relationship with the robotic devices, the impact of virtual reality, the use of social robots, the use of artificial intelligence, the integration between the artificial intelligence and virtual reality with the robotics, regulation issues) the element that showed the highest need for intervention was "the regulation issues".

Table 4. Output from the Likert question "Regarding the organizational aspects, what would you suggest to improve in terms of training and/or in-depth study in the field of ethics in robotic rehabilitation in the neurological field?".

Question	N(1)	N(2)	N(3)	N(4)	N(5)	N(6)	Score
The relationships with the robotic devices	2	6	4	27	40	76	5.01
The impact of the virtual reality	1	6	15	18	62	53	4.89
The use of social robots	3	7	16	18	64	47	4.77
The use of Artificial Intelligence	3	7	17	18	70	40	4.71
The integration between the artificial intelligence and virtual reality with the robotcs	4	5	14	18	68	46	4.80
The regulation issues	0	0	1	5	64	85	5.50

As for the Likert scale in Table 5 (question 10), all of the elements proposed showed that ethics was always considered a hindering issue. Among the elements proposed (the use of the robotics in general, the integration of robotics with artificial intelligence, the integration of robotics with virtual reality, the use of the social robot), the element that showed the greatest criticality regarding ethical aspects was "the use of the social robot".

Table 5. Output from the Likert question "Regarding the organizational aspects, do you think that ethical issues can hinder".

Question	N(1)	N(2)	N(3)	N(4)	N(5)	N(6)	Score
The use of the robotics in general	2	5	5	37	30	76	5.04
The integration of robotics with artificial intelligence	2	7	13	18	62	53	4.87
The integration of robotics with the virtual reality	4	6	15	19	54	57	4.83
The use of the social robot	0	0	1	11	11	132	5.77

Table 6 reports the output of the choice question related to the question "which aspect related to ethics worries you the most?" connected to the strategic items identified in [20].

Table 6. Output from the choice question "Which aspect related to ethics in Robotics worries you the most?".

Question	Number of Choices
Social cues	4
Privacy and data protection	2
Replacement	111
Autonomy	13
Trust and safety	5
Responsibility	10

The suggestion that had more answers was the replacement, with a percentage equal to 71.61%. Data security was viewed with less concern than all the other proposed aspects. The χ^2 applied to the frequencies of the choices showed a high significance ($p < 0.01$).

3.4. Feedback from the Participants

We analyzed the feedback obtained through open and graded questions. Figure 4 shows the high averaged values (score > 5) of the answers to the graded questions, highlighting a high degree of acceptance of the methodology in regard to all of the proposed parameters: reliability, practicality, clarity, usefulness, and potential. Furthermore, the Cronbach's α value of individual factors was assessed. It reported a score = 0.73, i.e., an encouraging level of reliability.

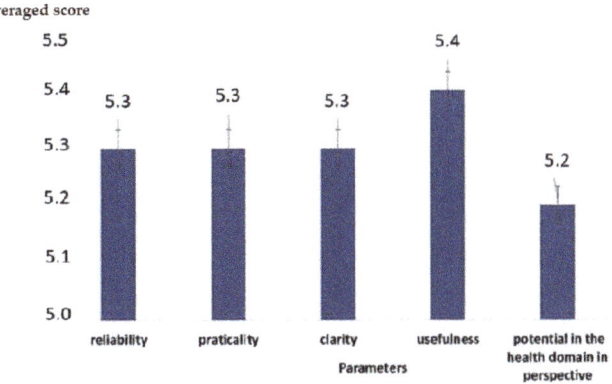

Figure 4. Averaged score for the different parameters proposed to assess the opinion of the participants.

The best six were selected based on a ranking considering both impact and significance.

They are reported in Box 1. The selection highlights: (a) a desire to further investigate ethical aspects and (b) concern about the impact of some of them.

Box 1. Selected open answers.

Comment
I am convinced that ethical aspects are given little space both to university courses and in the workplace. This applies to the entire healthcare sector and also to robotics
I think the introduction of social robots is rapidly approaching the era of robots with its own ethics. The problem is that if something is wrong in the design, there is a risk not only of malfunctions, but an impact on the patient's physical and mental health.
I fear that the introduction of robotics risks leading to a dehumanization of medical care and the ethical impacts are considerable. I am distinctly against it
I think that with the introduction of robotics in the medical field, the impact of ethics on the various professions will have to be seriously assessed, and consequently the ethical codes of the various professional orders will have to be heavily revised.
I think that in the future it will be necessary to work on many rehabilitation protocols and readjust them to the use of robots after heavy analysis of the impact of ethics.
I think that one of the critical aspect that we must consider is the equity in providing the robotic care. It should be avoided the discrimination of the less well-off

4. Discussion

Ethics have an important impact on the use of robotics in rehabilitation and assistance. [14,15] The implications are considerable and concern all aspects related to human replacement, data management and, as in the case of social robots, the programming of ethics itself. Regarding ethics programming, some studies have shown that programmers lack adequate cultural bases [17], which can create significant problems, including cybersecurity [12]. Regarding ethics in research and development, many studies, not all focused on the health domain, have identified some elements of concern (social cues, privacy and data protection, replacement, autonomy, trust and safety, and responsibility) [13,30]. In [30], it was highlighted how a population survey showed that the most critical was replacement.

In general, by adapting the model proposed in [12], it can be highlighted how the ethical issues can have a direct impact on both physical and psychological health (Figure 5).

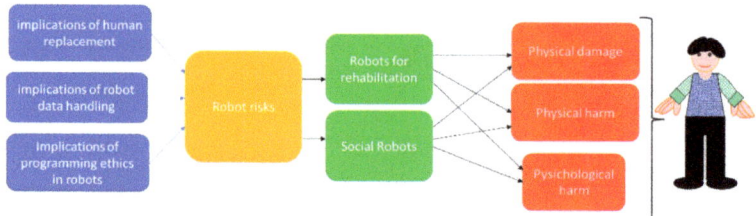

Figure 5. Model of impact of ethical issues.

The impact on both physical and mental health and on IT security makes it necessary to pay particular attention to ethics. This attention must start from the training processes during studies and continue in the workplace. Both the perceived level of knowledge in this area and the insiders' opinions need to be monitored. Recently, in line with our position, many studies are analysing the ethical problems in many areas of robotics [41,42] including the one we have taken into consideration [43].

Our study, focused on the health domain, proposed a survey on insiders with two polarities. The first consists of a point of view that deals with robotics and related technologies: (a) the training position during university studies and in the world of work, (b) the organizational aspects hindered by ethics and to be perfected in relation to ethics, and (c) aspects of ethics of concern. The second point of view consists of both structured and open-ended feedback on the proposed methodology. This study highlights an increase in mastery of ethical aspects in the workplace, a criticality in the regulatory aspects related to ethics and a major obstacle in social robotics. In line with the study conducted in [30], one of the aspects of greatest concern was considered to be the replacement of humans. We must consider that the study conducted in [30] was not focused on the health domain, but instead on service applications of robotics. Furthermore, ordinary citizens were included in this study, while in our study, insiders from the health domain were included who also expressed their perceptions on other issues such as training, organization, and needs for further study and obstacle. They also reported the positive feedback of high acceptance of the methodology with impressions in an open text form.

Our study is in line with other approaches in this field considering training [44]. The study reported in [44] considered the ethics in training, where despite a broad consensus on the ethical dimensions of the teaching profession, little is known about how teacher candidates are being prepared to face the ethical challenges of contemporary teaching. It presented the results of an international survey on ethics content and curriculum in initial teacher education involving five Organization for Economic Co-Operation and Development countries—the United States, England, Canada, Australia, and the Netherlands. Our study, as in [44], reiterates both the importance of training in ethics and the importance of surveys in these studies. Furthermore, our study provides, in a certain sense, a complementary result. While the study reported in [44] is focused on the role of trainers, our study is focused on those who participate as a learner in training courses in a sector where ethics has a particular impact.

Our study is also in line with what is highlighted in [45], where the importance of ethical aspects was addressed; it was highlighted that ethics is among the key aspects to be considered in the integration of robotics consensus (guidelines, health technology assessment, and consensus conferences). Indeed, at the Italian national Conference of consent in this field, through the activity of a dedicated working group [46], the following were highlighted: the important role ethics plays and specific recommendations on this issue, such as a stimulus for stakeholders and researchers, which we followed with the launch of this study. The state of the perception of ethics is as an obstacle on the part of insiders; this is in line with the results of the Likert questions reported in Table 5. Considering the above, the general added value of our study consists of a methodology, based on an electronic survey to investigate this issue, adapted to a category of insiders involved in interaction in the health domain.

From a more specific point of view, the study returns the following three added values:

The first added value is the electronic survey product which, although in a prototypal form, can also be investigated and used in future applications as a monitoring tool and by scientific societies.

The second added value is represented by the first outcome of quantitative and indicative data from the study.

The third added value is represented by both structured feedback and observations from patients.

Limitations

The first two limitations are those typical of the electronic surveys, as those ones indicated in national studies based on these tools [47], i.e., the willingness and the type of administration, that includes the participants in the study with a "fishing on the pile procedure", that we strained to compensate for by designing and applying a robust statistic.

A third limitation is that the survey is a prototype. It can be improved through the intervention of scientific societies to include other professionals, and then used in consensus integration initiatives, such as in consensus conferences [45,46].

5. Conclusions

Ethics represents a key aspect for the introduction of robotics in the world of rehabilitation and assistance. The study focused on the category of health domain insiders.

A targeted survey was developed on this issue. This survey made it possible to obtain various outcomes. First, the study reported both the state of academic training on this topic and the knowledge subsequently integrated into the world of work. Second, the study highlighted, in terms of perceptions, strong criticalities of the regulatory aspects regarding organizational aspects and strong ethical obstacles on the introduction of social robots. Third, among the aspects of concern the most relevant was the replacement of humans with robots. The study also reported a high acceptance of participants and suggests future developments in these areas in collaboration with scientific societies.

Author Contributions: Conceptualization, D.G. and G.M.; methodology, D.G.; software, D.G., A.P. and P.M.; validation, All; formal analysis, D.G.; investigation, All; resources, All; data curation, D.G.; writing—original draft preparation, D.G.; writing—review and editing, D.G., G.M., A.P. and P.M.; visualization, A.P. and P.M.; supervision, D.G. and G.M.; project administration, Not Applicable; funding acquisition, Not Applicable. All authors have read and agreed to the published version of the manuscript.

Funding: The APC was funded by the corresponding author.

Institutional Review Board Statement: Not applicable.

Informed Consent Statement: Not applicable.

Data Availability Statement: Not applicable.

Conflicts of Interest: The authors declare no conflict of interest.

References

1. Dolic, Z.; Castro, R.; Moarcas, A. Robots in Healthcare: A Solution or a Problem? Study for the Committee on Environment, Public Health, and Food Safety. Luxembourg: Policy Department for Economic, Scientific and Quality of Life Policies, European Parliament. 2019. Available online: https://www.europarl.europa.eu/RegData/etudes/IDAN/2019/638391/IPOL_IDA(2019)638391_EN.pdf (accessed on 25 November 2021).
2. Boldrini, P.; Bonaiuti, D.; Mazzoleni, S.; Posteraro, F. Rehabilitation assisted by robotic and electromechanical devices for people with neurological disabilities: Contributions for the preparation of a national conference in Italy. *Eur. J. Phys. Rehabil. Med.* **2021**, *57*, 458–459. [CrossRef] [PubMed]
3. Giansanti, D. The Rehabilitation and the Robotics: Are They Going Together Well? *Healthcare* **2021**, *9*, 26. [CrossRef] [PubMed]
4. Sheridan, T.B. A review of recent research in social robotics. *Curr. Opin. Psychol.* **2020**, *36*, 7–12. [CrossRef]
5. Lötsch, J.; Kringel, D.; Ultsch, A. Explainable Artificial Intelligence (XAI) in Biomedicine: Making AI Decisions Trustworthy for Physicians and Patients. *BioMedInformatics* **2022**, *2*, 1–17. [CrossRef]
6. Datta, A.; Matlock, M.K.; Le Dang, N.; Moulin, T.; Woeltje, K.F.; Yanik, E.L.; Swamidass, S.J. 'Black Box' to 'Conversational' Machine Learning: Ondansetron Reduces Risk of Hospital-Acquired Venous Thromboembolism. *IEEE J. Biomed. Health Inform.* **2021**, *25*, 2204–2214. [CrossRef] [PubMed]
7. Datta, A.; Flynn, N.R.; Barnette, D.A.; Woeltje, K.F.; Miller, G.P.; Swamidass, S.J. Machine learning liver-injuring drug interactions with non-steroidal anti-inflammatory drugs (NSAIDs) from a retrospective electronic health record (EHR) cohort. *PLoS Comput. Biol.* **2021**, *17*, e1009053. [CrossRef] [PubMed]
8. Giovagnoli, M.R.; Giansanti, D. Artificial Intelligence in Digital Pathology: What Is the Future? Part 1: From the Digital Slide Onwards. *Healthcare* **2021**, *9*, 858. [CrossRef] [PubMed]
9. Giansanti, D.; Di Basilio, F. The Artificial Intelligence in Digital Radiology: Part 1: The Challenges, Acceptance and Consensus. *Healthcare* **2022**, *10*, 509. [CrossRef] [PubMed]
10. D'Antonoli, T.A. Ethical considerations for artificial intelligence: An overview of the current radiology landscape. *Diagn. Interv. Radiol.* **2020**, *26*, 504–511.
11. Banks, J. The Human Touch: Practical and Ethical Implications of Putting AI and Robotics to Work for Patients. *IEEE Pulse.* **2018**, *9*, 15–18. [CrossRef]
12. Fosch-Villaronga, E.; Mahler, T. Safety and robots: Strengthening the link between cybersecurity and safety in the context of care robots. *Comput. Law Secur. Rev.* **2021**, *41*, 105528. [CrossRef]
13. Stahl, B.C.; Coeckelbergh, M. Ethics of healthcare robotics: Towards responsible research and innovation. *Robot. Auton. Syst.* **2016**, *86*, 152–161. [CrossRef]
14. Datteri, E. Predicting the long-term effects of human robot interaction: A reflection on responsibility in medical robotics. *Sci. Eng. Ethics* **2013**, *19*, 139–160. [CrossRef]
15. Iosa, M.; Morone, G.; Cherubini, A.; Paolucci, S. The Three Laws of Neurorobotics: A Review on What Neurorehabilitation Robots Should Do for Patients and Clinicians. *J. Med. Biol Eng.* **2016**, *36*, 1–11. [CrossRef] [PubMed]
16. Morone, G. Robots for stroke rehabilitation: Not all that glitters is gold. *Funct Neurol.* **2019**, *34*, 5–6. [PubMed]

17. Gordon, J.S. Building moral robots: Ethical pitfalls and challenges. *Sci. Eng. Ethics* **2020**, *26*, 141–157. [CrossRef]
18. Coeckelbergh, M. Human development or human enhancement? A methodological reflection on capabilities and the evaluation of information technologies. *Ethics Inf. Technol.* **2011**, *13*, 81–92. [CrossRef]
19. Coeckelbergh, M. Are emotional robots deceptive? *IEEE Trans. Affect. Comput.* **2012**, *3*, 388–393. [CrossRef]
20. Coeckelbergh, M. E-care as craftsmanship: Virtuous work, skilled engagement, and information technology in health care. *Med. Health Care Philos.* **2013**, *16*, 807–816. [CrossRef]
21. Coeckelbergh, M. Good healthcare is in the "how": The quality of care, the role of machines, and the need for new skills. In *Machine Medical Ethics*; van Rysewyk, S.P., Pontier, M., Eds.; Springer: Berlin/Heidelberg, Germany, 2015; pp. 33–48.
22. Decker, M.; Fleischer, T. Contacting the brain—aspects of a technology assessment of neural implants. *Biotechnol. J.* **2008**, *3*, 1502–1510. [CrossRef]
23. Sharkey, A.; Sharkey, N. Granny and the robots: Ethical issues in robot care for the elderly. *Ethics Inform. Technol.* **2010**, *14*, 27–40. [CrossRef]
24. Sparrow, R.; Sparrow, L. In the hands of machines? The future of aged care. *Minds Mach.* **2006**, *16*, 141–161. [CrossRef]
25. Whitby, B. Do you want a robot lover? In *Robot. Ethics: The Ethical and Social Implications of Robotics*; Lin, P., Abney, K., Bekey, G.A., Eds.; MIT Press: Cambridge, MA, USA, 2011; pp. 233–249.
26. Wallach, W.; Allen, C. *Moral Machines: Teaching Robots Right from Wrong*; Oxford University Press: Oxford, UK, 2010.
27. Anderson, M.; Anderson, S.L. *Machine Ethics*; Cambridge University Press: Cambridge, MA, USA, 2011.
28. Gunkel, D.J.; Bryson, J. The machine as moral agent and patient. *Philos. Technol.* **2014**, *27*, 5–142. [CrossRef]
29. Anderson, S.L. Machine metaethics. In *Machine Ethics*; Anderson, M., Anderson, S.L., Eds.; Cambridge University Press: Cambridge, MA, USA, 2011; pp. 21–27.
30. Etemad-Sajadi, R.; Soussan, A.; Schöpfer, T. How Ethical Issues Raised by Human-Robot Interaction can Impact the Intention to use the Robot? *Int. J. Soc. Robot.* **2022**, *13*, 1–13. [CrossRef]
31. Beer, J.M.; Prakash, A.; Mitzner, T.L.; Rogers, W.A. Understanding Robot Acceptance. *Ga. Inst. Technol.* **2011**, 1–45. Available online: https://smartech.gatech.edu/bitstream/handle/1853/39672/HFA-TR-1103-RobotAcceptance.pdf (accessed on 10 March 2022).
32. Gefen, D.; Karahanna, E.; Straub, D. Trust and TAM in online shopping: An integrated model. *MIS Q* **2003**, *27*, 51–90. [CrossRef]
33. *European Union's Convention on Roboethics*; European Union: Maastricht, The Netherlands, 2010.
34. Lin, P.; Abney, K.; Bekey, G.A. *Robot. Ethics: The Ethical and Social Implications of Robotics*; The MIT Press: Cambridge, MA, USA, 2014.
35. Graeff, T.R.; Harmon, S. Collecting and using personal data: Consumers' awareness and concerns. *J. Consum Mark.* **2002**, *19*, 302–318. [CrossRef]
36. Nizamis, K.; Athanasiou, A.; Almpani, S.; Dimitrousis, C.; Astaras, A. Converging Robotic Technologies in Targeted Neural Rehabilitation: A Review of Emerging Solutions and Challenges. *Sensors* **2021**, *21*, 2084. [CrossRef]
37. Obermeyer, Z.; Powers, B.; Vogeli, C.; Mullainathan, S. Dissecting racial bias in an algorithm used to manage the health of populations. *Science* **2019**, *366*, 447–453. [CrossRef]
38. Available online: https://forms.office.com/Pages/ResponsePage.aspx?id=DQSIkWdsW0yxEjajBLZtrQAAAAAAAAAAZAAOUXdFhUM1UxU0VDMEM0ODYyQUZXWTYzMU1WOTJYSS4u (accessed on 10 March 2022).
39. Available online: https://drive.google.com/file/d/1rKPyhpYc9ThmhURJEfr2WiLOuZ9FUi86/view?usp=sharing (accessed on 10 March 2022).
40. Available online: https://www.surveymonkey.com/mp/likert-scale/ (accessed on 10 March 2022).
41. Eiben, Á.E.; Ellers, J.; Meynen, G.; Nyholm, S. Robot Evolution: Ethical Concerns. *Front. Robot. AI* **2021**, *8*, 744590. [CrossRef]
42. Kok, B.C.; Soh, H. Trust in Robots: Challenges and Opportunities. *Curr. Robot. Rep.* **2020**, *1*, 297–309. [CrossRef] [PubMed]
43. Cornet, G. Robot companions and ethics a pragmatic approach of ethical design. *J. Int. Bioethique* **2013**, *24*, 49–58, 179–180. [CrossRef] [PubMed]
44. Maxwell, B.; Tremblay-Laprise, A.A.; Filion, M.; Boon, H.; Daly, C.; van den Hoven, M.; Heilbronn, R.; Lenselink, M.; Walters, S. A five-country survey on ethics education in preservice teaching programs. *J. Teach. Educ.* **2016**, *67*, 135–151. [CrossRef]
45. Maccioni, G.; Ruscitto, S.; Gulino, R.A.; Giansanti, D. Opportunities and Problems of the Consensus Conferences in the Care Robotics. *Healthcare* **2021**, *9*, 1624. [CrossRef] [PubMed]
46. SIMFER; SIRN. Documento Definitivo di Consenso a Cura della Giuria della Consensus Conference CICERONE. Available online: https://www.simfer.it/wp-content/uploads/doc_vari/2022_Doc_Finale_ConsensusConferenceRoboticaCICERONE/CONSENSUSCICERONE-DOCUMENTOFINALEDEF.-con-licenza-2.pdf (accessed on 10 March 2022).
47. Choi, H.; Jeong, G. Characteristics of the Measurement Tools for Assessing Health Information-Seeking Behaviors in Nationally Representative Surveys: Systematic Review. *J. Med. Internet Res.* **2021**, *23*, e27539. [CrossRef] [PubMed]

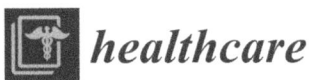 healthcare

Opinion

Opportunities and Problems of the Consensus Conferences in the *Care Robotics*

Giovanni Maccioni [1], Selene Ruscitto [2], Rosario Alfio Gulino [2] and Daniele Giansanti [1,*]

[1] Centro Nazionale per le Tecnologie Innovative in Sanità Pubblica, Istituto Superiore di Sanità, 00161 Rome, Italy; giovanni.maccioni@iss.it
[2] Faculty of Engineering, Tor Vergata University, 00133 Rome, Italy; seleneruscitto@hotmail.com (S.R.); rosario.gulino.uni.tv@hotmail.com (R.A.G.)
* Correspondence: Daniele.giansanti@iss.it

Abstract: Care robots represent an opportunity for the *health domain*. The use of these devices has important implications. They can be used in surgical operating rooms in important and delicate clinical interventions, in motion, in training-and-simulation, and cognitive and rehabilitation processes. They are involved in continuous processes of evolution in technology and clinical practice. Therefore, the introduction into routine clinical practice is difficult because this needs the stability and the standardization of processes. *The agreement tools*, in this case, are of primary importance for the clinical acceptance and introduction. The opinion focuses on the *Consensus Conference* tool and: (a) highlights its potential in the field; (b) explores the state of use; (c) detects the peculiarities and problems (d) expresses ideas on how improve its diffusion.

Keywords: e-health; medical devices; m-health; rehabilitation; robotics; organization models; artificial intelligence; electronic surveys; social robots; collaborative robots; cyber risk; informatics; consensus conference; acceptance; clinical acceptance

Citation: Maccioni, G.; Ruscitto, S.; Gulino, R.A.; Giansanti, D. Opportunities and Problems of the Consensus Conferences in the *Care Robotics*. *Healthcare* **2021**, *9*, 1624. https://doi.org/10.3390/healthcare9121624

Academic Editor: Francesco Faita

Received: 15 September 2021
Accepted: 20 November 2021
Published: 24 November 2021

Publisher's Note: MDPI stays neutral with regard to jurisdictional claims in published maps and institutional affiliations.

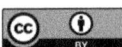

Copyright: © 2021 by the authors. Licensee MDPI, Basel, Switzerland. This article is an open access article distributed under the terms and conditions of the Creative Commons Attribution (CC BY) license (https://creativecommons.org/licenses/by/4.0/).

1. Introduction

The Policy Department for Economic, Scientific and Quality of Life Policies of the European Parliament identified the most interesting applications of the care robots (CR)s [1] divided into four groups:
- Robotic surgery
- Care and socially assistive robots
- Rehabilitation systems
- Training for health and care workers

1.1. The Care Robots: Advantages and Disadvantages

The discussion on the merits and demerits of robots is a current topic both in the world of industry and consumption [2,3] and in the *health domain* [4]. Employing robots in a *health domain* brings innumerable benefits and is equally advantageous for both healthcare providers and patients.

Robotic surgery, for example, has reduced the risk of infection, the blood loss, and improves the recovery time for the patients. The use of robotics in rehabilitation and assistance improves the care and decreases the professionals' workload. The robots in the *health domain* near always are practical, useful, effective, and tireless.

All this makes the use of robots particularly useful in the following applications [4]:

Surgeries—Robot-assisted surgeries are reliable, precise, flexible, and practical. They allow "minimally invasive" surgical actions.

Clinical Training—Clinical training robots are realistic simulation devices using also haptic systems very useful in the training.

Prescription/Dispensing—These robots can both dispense medicine at a very high speed and accuracy and similarly handle sensitive liquids or viscous materials.

Care/Services—These robots aid both to perform daily activities (for example moving, transport) and daily check-ups (like temperature, blood sugar, pressure).

Disinfection and Sanitation—These specialized robots carry important routine actions in the *health domain*, such as the air circulating and surface disinfection process.

Telepresence—They are telemedicine robots, designed to interact with the patient from remote locations. They can be also used in domotics.

Logistic robots—The logistics robots equipped with navigation systems perform basic tasks such as moving lunches or medications.

Rehabilitation Robots and Nursing/Assistance Robots are also other important robots generating significant interest.

While there are innumerable benefits of employing robots to run tasks in the *health domain*, there are probabilities of faults. There is always some scope for human error or mechanical failure with these advanced robots. A single mechanical fault can cause physical damages/harms, psychological harm (for example the social robots) or even death. Another major disadvantage is the cost factor. The use of surgical robots or robots for rehabilitation and assistance is limited to the developed countries. Other problems are represented by the strong impact and implications of the ethics in this field [5,6].

1.2. The Strong Need of the Agreement Initiatives in Care Robotics

CRs are taking on an increasingly important role in the *health domain*. A simple search on Pubmed with key (*robot [title/abstract]*) [7] shows that to date (07/09/2021) 22,776 studies referring in some way to CRs are accessible in this Database. A total of 8693 (equal to 38.1%) of them have been published between January 2019 to date. There is no doubt that the CR sector is growing rapidly. The CR sector is a highly scientifically innovative sector subject to continuous research developments and innovations.

Therefore, the standardization processes that lead to routine use in the clinical setting are in a state of constant chase. National and international regulations (governing development and certification processes and use in the clinical setting) are often of a general nature or not specifically designed for devices subject to continuous technological innovation.

Think, for example, the cybersecurity implications for these systems [8,9].

Furthermore, the organizational models for using CRs are different depending on the application. They differ not only from country to country, but also between regions and areas of the same country, or among application regimes (e.g., public, or private). This makes the results of scientific research (revisions for example) not immediately applicable or translatable, precisely because they may also depend on the organizational model where they have been applied. For example, Italy has a regionalized *health domain* organization, with different delivery methods, depending by region and on whether it is a public or private service provider [10].

Tackling the issue of acceptance (through proper tools is mandatory) into the clinical routine is a hot and current issue, with several implications of various fields, such as ethics, safety, cybersecurity, laws, and policy. It is a multidimensional problem in the *health domain* with several variables (e.g., the evolution of research, the regulatory framework, the organizational model, the acceptance and opinion of insiders, the cost-effectiveness, the training).

An approach in this area certainly starts from evidence-based medicine (EBM) and then must use agreement tools.

The EBM [11–13] aims to guarantee all patients the same quality, efficiency, and effectiveness of intervention, overcoming some limitations of the individual experience of clinicians. In recent years, the progress achieved by research allows for the constant and updated production of new knowledge. Useful tools for disseminating knowledge have been developed such as *systematic reviews, meta-analyses, reviews of literature, decision-making systems based on formal models*. Since the 1980s, to respond even more precisely and punctually to these knowledge transfer needs and to produce useful recommendations for guiding clinical practice, *"guidelines"* (GL) [14], *"technology assessment"* (TA) reports [15–17] and *"consensus conferences* [18,19] are born. The *Consensus Conferences* (CC)s are tools, allowing, through a road map (based on a formally shared and structured process), an agreement on a topic. The purpose of the CC is to produce evidence-based recommendations, useful to assist operators and patients in a multidimensional domain.

1.3. The Purpose and Structure of the Study

The goal of the *opinion* is to explore the use of the CCs on the CRs, identifying the state of application, the opportunities and-problems that have emerged, and providing reflections to scholars and stakeholders.

The study is organized into two sections plus the introduction (Section 1) and the conclusions (Section 4). Section 2 recalls, based on a brief review of the scientific literature, the relevance of the CC tool. Section 3 analyses (a) the state of application of this tool in Care Robotics. (b) The opportunities and-problems that have emerged. (c) The aspects that have been little or no dealt with.

2. The Consensus Conferences: Brief Reminder and Relevance

The purpose of a CC is to produce evidence-based recommendations useful to assist operators and patients in a *multidimensional domain*. The CC agreement tool [18,19], can use, the output of both TA Reports (TR)s studies and GLs. However, it can also use other tools for monitoring or collecting opinions, such as *surveys* and *focus groups*. GLs and TRs are analysed by experts recruited for the CC. Compared to other tools, the CC allows, thanks to the possibility of breaking down the problem into specific questions, to share and precisely clarify the points on which there is greater uncertainty, thus laying the right premises to obtain targeted and precise answers, consult databases in a specific way, excluding that little or irrelevant part of the literature. The US National Institutes of Health established the Consensus Development Program in 1977 [20] with the aim of providing independent, impartial, and evidence-based assessments of complex medical issues, developing the consensus conference tool for the first time. The method, modified several times over the years, involves the interfacing of different actors and phases. In addition, other nations developed similar methods [20], as for example the France [21]. In Italy the Istituto Superiore di Sanità (The Italian NIH) produced a Manual for the CCs in 2008 [13] and followed several CCs as.

2.1. An Organizing Committee Starts the Work of the Conference

One or more subjects interested in the chosen topic can play this role, including: institutions, scientific societies, experts in the sector in question, patient associations or their families. The a priori presence of a public institutional subject (for example in Italy the Istituto Superiore di Sanità, the Italian National Institute of Health) could benefit the entire process. The latter, as a neutral figure, would have the possibility of intervening in resolving any conflicting opinions of the interested parties in various capacities. Furthermore, this would favour the dissemination and application on the national territory of the produced recommendations. There are several actors in a CC.

In addition to develop the conference, the *Organizing Committee* (OC) selects the members of both the *Technical-Scientific Committee* (TSC), the *Jury Panel* (JP), the experts of the *working groups* (WG)s and provide them with methodological support together with the TSC.

2.2. The Working Groups (WG) Plays a Fundamental Role

The principal question, to be answered by the CC, will be divided into articulated *sub-questions*. Each *sub-question* will be assigned to a specific WG.

These are composed of experts with very specific skills in relation to the subject examined. These are multidisciplinary groups, which, are required, (starting from the critical analysis and evaluation of the available scientific evidence), to summarize the latter and prepare reports with which to expose the data to the JP. In robotics, as in other fields, the success of a CC depends on how the *sub-questions* assigned to each *WG* are articulated.

3. The Consensus Conferences and the Care Robots: State of Application, Opportunities, and Problems

The sector of the CRs has experienced a significant and constant increase in recent years. However, there is a strong inhomogeneity in the criteria for clinical use, as well as in the evaluation of the outcomes. The CC tool could be greatly useful.

3.1. The State of Application

We investigated the application status of the CC. In line with this type of contribution, we did a e search on Pubmed with the key: (consensus conference) AND (robot [title/abstract])

The search [22] returns 17 results [23–39].

After an analysis of the records, 4 studies were discarded because they were not completely relevant. The 13 remaining references are the following [23–26,28,30,32–36,38,39].

Another search "with the key: consensus conference" shows [40] 21.779 results.

Specific search in the field of the application but without referring to robots returns:

- With the key: (consensus conference) AND (surgery) [Title/Abstract]) [41] 1.676 results.
- With the key: (consensus conference) AND (rehabilitation) [Title/Abstract]) [42] 372 results.
- With the key: (consensus conference) AND (assistance) [Title/Abstract]) [43] 94 results.
- With the key: (consensus conference) AND (training) [Title/Abstract]) [44] 800 results.

The results obtained in [22] is equal to a percentage ranging from 1.01% (in the case of surgery) up to 18.09% (in the case of assistance).

Table 1 highlights the detected sectors [23–26,28,30,32–36,38,39] dedicated to rehabilitation, diagnostics, therapy, and surgery.

Table 1. Application of the consensus conference in robotics.

Reference	Application
[23–25]	Robotics in neurorehabilitation
[26]	Robots used in transcranial magnetic stimulation
[28]	Training in robot-assisted Surgery
[30]	Robotics on laparoscopic liver resection.
[32–34]	Robot assisted radical cystectomy
[35,36]	Robot assisted radical prostatectomy
[38]	Robotic pelvic surgery
[39]	Robots used in simulation environments

Appendix A.1, in Appendix A, reports the highlights from studies in Table 1 in details.

3.2. Opportunities and Emerging Problems

From a general point of view, it emerges (Table 1 and Appendix A.1) that the CC tool is currently used in the context of the CRs. CCs were used in all the applications in [1], except for Social Robots, probably because this type of CR is the most recent and is the one most subject to technological updating. The studies also highlight that the CCs have been an important opportunity for the connection between experts operating in various fields, from bioengineering up to clinics. Each CC, reported in the Table 1, Appendix A.1, faces the robotics in a highly specific clinical question; this allows experts to better focus on a question and investigate the problem in more detail. The CC deals with a specific topic, as for example [23] *the robot* in *neurological rehabilitation (a specific sector of rehabilitation)*. Again, for example, the *surgical robot* in *Radical Cystectomy (a specific surgical sector)* [32]. In some cases, the CR is not the direct focus of the CC. Nevertheless, its important role and its innovation is faced [26,30]. Among the methodological tools used in the CCs, we also find, not only the review, but also the surveys and the focus groups [26,32–34]. It also emerges that the CCs involved scientific societies locally, or regionally (e.g., Europe, Asia). In the articles in Table 1, however, the activities of the CCs are only partially reported. Furthermore, it is not possible to make a constructive comparison between the various studies. The contents relating to the total output of the CC are therefore not available on Pubmed. Probably because the final documents, when available, have been disseminated through different editorial tools (e.g., national monographs or by scientific societies or by sponsoring bodies or guarantor bodies). In consideration of the previous point, we should consider that the *medical knowledge* must be made also by accessing and monitoring the web of the scientific societies/associations (sponsoring or supporting the initiatives) or of the guarantor bodies. This makes the work of experts and researchers difficult to carry out with obvious difficulties due to both the fragmentation and the relative retrieval of documentation. The search on the Web, confirms this. It highlights how the information on the CCs is distributed and spread over various resources. It can be found, partially, dynamically updated, on the websites of the sponsoring scientific societies [45], on the website of the Guarantor Body [46], or on other national databases [47]. We have also extended a web search to technologies that can somehow intersect with CRs. We have noticed that Assistive Technologies can intersect with the CRs, starting from the definition [48,49]. Also, in this case, CCs are reported on the web [50,51]. Surely, these latter considerations, on the information availability [45–51], highlight how the attention must also be shifted outside of Pubmed, monitoring, and tracking the web of the scientific societies, associations and guarantor bodies.

3.3. Aspects Not Adequately Explored in the Consensus Conferences in Robotics

Based on what emerged from the research in the literature there are aspects that have not been adequately explored on the CC in this sector. Indeed, two further issues need to be deepened for the CRs (compared to other biomedical technologies).

1. *The implications with ethics, regulatory aspects and in the new emerging risks (for example Cybersecurity)*. Ethics has an important role and a peculiarity on the CRs, such as on the SRs. The ethical issues on CRs have identified two *macro-sectors* [5,6]. The first *macro-sector* is the ethics in a responsible research and innovation [5]. The second *macro-sector* is the ethics problem encountered while building moral CRs [6]. There are *shadows* in EU Medical Device (MD) regulations [52]. *First*, they focus a lot on manufacturers and little on recipients/users. *Second*, the intended use and certification [53], must be aligned, and this is not always easily feasible in the field of the medical devices; for this reason the *health domain* supervisory systems are always active with monitoring actions. There are limits in the application of specific Cyb certifications. They are voluntary, as in the case of the Cybersecurity ACT [54]. The CRs would need an ad hoc regulatory framework, in consideration of the peculiarities [8].
2. *How to organize the WGs considering the peculiarity of the CR*. The organization of the WGs has a basic importance. The principal question, to be answered by the CC, is, indeed, divided into articulated sub-questions. In robotics, as in other fields, the success of a CC depends on how the *sub-questions* assigned to each WG are articulated.

The key queries that a CC must answer in a specific clinical application of specific CRs, also considering the previous point, (based on current scientific knowledge and experience gained in the recent years), are the following:

- Definitions and classification criteria for the devices based on the intended use.
- Indications on the specific clinical use of devices in clinical applications.
- Scientific References and consolidated experience for the development of the CRs.
- Organizational contexts and changes in the workflow.

- Regulatory framework (including the cybersecurity) and ethical issues for the devices.

The literature research did not provide always-clear suggestions on the WGs organization. However, in [47] we can find a proposal of WGs for a specific CC in neurorehabilitation, which also considered some of the above listed issues. This is useful also to stimulate other CCs.

Based on this and the above considerations our *opinion* is that a set of *WGs* can be defined as in Appendix A.2 (Appendix A), for example, for a generic CC raging from robots for neurosurgery up to social robotics.

4. Conclusions

The sector of the CRs has experienced a significant and constant increase in recent years. However, there are strong inhomogeneities in the criteria for clinical use, as well as in the evaluation of their outcomes. The national and international bodies must contribute to concretize the efforts of national and international research. They must make available through consensus initiatives, their skills in the technical–scientific–regulatory field. The agreement tools are therefore strategic for this. The CCs are agreement tools, allowing, through a road map [18–21] (based on a formally shared and structured process), an agreement on a complex and articulated topic. They produce evidence-based recommendations, useful to assist operators and patients in a multidimensional domain. They have a strong potential on CRs because they can focus on a specific task (e.g., a specific clinical application of a specific CR), stress it, and considers a large set of implications. We first investigated the use of CCs in care robotics.

The analysis of the scientific literature has highlighted some *lights* and *shadows*.

Among the lights, we highlight the following: (a) the CC tool, [23–26,28,30,32–36,38,39], was used in the fields of *rehabilitation, diagnostics, therapy, and surgery*, on all applications of consolidated CRs [1], (with the exception of Social Robots, which are still subject to technological stabilization processes). (b) The CCs were the opportunity to: (1) bring together national and international experts from different cultural backgrounds in national and international meetings, (1) make them work around a structured and wide-ranging review process. This guarantees a broad consensus. (b)There has been a wide involvement of national and international scientific societies dealing with the application. (c) The methodologies to be used have been individuated. In addition to the consolidated reviews of the literature, the methodologies that can operate on the territory and on the groups involved were also indicated (for example questionnaires and focus groups).

Among the *shadows*, we highlight the following: (a) the studies available on the leading *health domain* databases (e.g., Pubmed) do not report the definitive documents but only partial considerations. Information is scattered on the networks, for example, partially available on the webs of the *scientific societies/associations* sponsoring the initiatives or of the guarantor bodies. This makes the work of experts and researchers difficult to carry. (b) The implications with ethics must be deepened. Ethics has an important role and a peculiarity on CRs, ranging from the ethical issues in research and innovation [5] up to ethics problems encountered while building moral CRs [6]. (c) The limits of the EU Medical Device (MD) regulations [52] must be considered, as: (1) the regulations focus a lot on manufacturers and little on recipients/users. (2) The intended use and certification [53], sometimes, are difficult to align. (d) The problems of the new emerging risk of cybersecurity must be carefully considered. The certification on the cybersecurity, according to the Cybersecurity ACT [54], is voluntary. Therefore, CCs must express clear suggestions for this. (e) It is not easy to find clear indications on how organizing *WGs* in a CC. The organization of the *WGs* has a basic importance. In robotics, as in other disciplines, the success of a CC depends on how the WGs are articulated.

Final Reflection

There is an increasing policy interest in renovating healthcare in a way comparable to how robotics transformed the industry, in terms of augmented productivity and resource effectiveness and productivity.

The introduction of these systems in clinical practice, and more generally in the *health domain*, requires great efforts of agreement through appropriate tools that consider all dimensions of the problems (e.g., clinical, regulatory and cost-effectiveness). In our study, we investigated the use, criticalities, and opportunities of the CCs.

International stakeholders need to undertake:

- Initiatives of greater diffusion of the methodology through tools that give it wide visibility.
- Census and categorization of the past and ongoing CCs.
- Coordination and initiation of CC programs at both national and international level involving the greatest number of experts.

Author Contributions: Conceptualization, D.G.; methodology, D.G.; software, All; validation, All; formal analysis, All; investigation, All; resources, All; data curation, All; writing—original draft preparation, D.G.; writing—review and editing, D.G., R.A.G., G.M., S.R.; visualization, All; supervision, D.G.; project administration, D.G. and R.A.G.; All authors have read and agreed to the published version of the manuscript.

Funding: This research received no external funding.

Institutional Review Board Statement: Not applicable.

Informed Consent Statement: Not applicable.

Data Availability Statement: Not applicable.

Conflicts of Interest: The authors declare no conflict of interest.

Appendix A

Appendix A.1. Summary of the Highlights from the Studies from Pubmed

Topic	Summary
Robotics in Neurorehabilitation	The general purpose of the CC was the elaboration of recommendations relating to various aspects of the use of robotic technologies and of all electromechanical devices used in the clinical rehabilitation centers to optimize rehabilitation treatment for people with disabilities of neurological origin: indications and modalities of use, organization, training of professionals, without neglecting the important ethical, legal and regulatory aspects.
Robots used in Transcranial magnetic stimulation	The CC intended to update the ten-year-old safety guidelines for the application of transcranial magnetic stimulation (TMS) in research and clinical settings. Therefore, only emerging and new issues are covered in detail, leaving still valid the 2009 recommendations. New issues discussed in detail from the meeting up to April 2020 are safety issues of recently developed stimulation devices and pulse configurations; duties and responsibility of device makers; novel scenarios of TMS applications such as in the neuroimaging context or imaging-guided and robot-guided.
Training in Robot-assisted Surgery	This CC established a basis for bringing surgical robotic training out of the operating room by seeking input and consensus across surgical specialties for an objective, validated, and standardised training programme with transparent, metric-based training outcomes. The panel achieved consensus that standardised international training pathways should be the basis for a structured, validated, replicable, and certified approach to implementation of robotic technology.
Robotics on laparoscopic liver resection	The CC dealt with the robotics in laparoscopic liver resection. The first Asiatic Pacific CC on laparoscopic liver resection was held in July 2016 in Hong Kong. A group of expert liver surgeons with experience laparoscopic hepatectomy convened to formulate recommendations on the role and perspective of laparoscopic liver resection for primary liver cancer
Robot assisted Radical Cystectomy	The CC faced the robotics in Radical cystectomy (RC). RC is associated with frequent morbidity and prolonged length of stay (LOS) irrespective of surgical approach. Increasing evidence from colorectal surgery indicates that minimally invasive surgery and enhanced recovery programmes (ERPs) can reduce surgical morbidity and LOS. ERPs are now recognised as an important component of surgical management for RC. However, there is comparatively little evidence for ERPs after robot-assisted radical cystectomy (RARC). Consensus was reached in multiple areas of an ERP for RARC. The key principles include patient education, optimisation of nutrition, RARC approach, standardised anaesthetic, analgesic, and antiemetic regimens, and early mobilisation.
Robot assisted Radical Prostatectomy	The CC faced the Radical retropubic prostatectomy (RRP). RRP has long been the most common surgical technique used to treat clinically localized prostate cancer (PCa). More recently, robot-assisted radical prostatectomy (RARP) has been gaining increasing acceptance among patients and urologists, and it has become the dominant technique in the United States despite a paucity of prospective studies or randomized trials supporting its superiority over RRP. RARP may offer advantages in postoperative recovery of urinary continence and erectile function, although there are methodological limitations in most studies to date and a need for well-controlled comparative outcomes studies of radical prostatectomy surgery following best practice guidelines. Surgeon experience and institutional volume of procedures strongly predict better outcomes in all relevant domains. Available evidence suggests that RARP is a valuable therapeutic option for clinically localized PCa. Further research is needed to clarify the actual role of RARP in patients with locally advanced disease.
Robotic Pelvic surgery	The CC faced the robotics in Pelvic Surgery. At the Meeting held in Brescia in June 2007, the participants focused on the role of robotic surgery in pelvic operations surgery for malignancy including prostate, rectal, uterine, and cervical carcinoma. All members of the interdisciplinary panel were asked to define the role of robotic surgery in prostate, rectal, and uterine carcinoma. All key statements were reformulated until a consensus within the group was achieved. Evidences highlighted that while robotic prostatectomy has become the most widely accepted method of prostatectomy, robotic hysterectomy and proctectomy remain far less widely accepted. The theoretical benefits of the increased degrees of freedom and three-dimensional visualization may be outweighed in these areas by the loss of haptic feedback, increased operative times, and increased cost.
Robots used in simulation environments	The CC focused on Simulation environments. Simulation is currently used to model teamwork-communication skills for disaster management and critical events, but little research or evidence exists to show that simulation improves disaster response or facilitates intersystem or interagency com-munication. The CC highlighted that simulation ranges from the use of standardized patient encounters to robot-mannequins to computerized virtual environments. As such, the field of simulation covers a broad range of interactions, from patient-physician encounters to that of the interfaces between larger systems and agencies.

A.2. The WGs Architecture for a Consensus Conference on the CRs in a Defined Clinical Application

WG	Objective
"Device classification based on the intended use"	To collect documentation on the classification issues based on the specific intended use
"The specific clinical use of the CR".	To collect evidences/documentation on the clinical applications
"Models of use and research directions".	To collect evidences/documentation on the model of use and the research directions
"Organizational models and work flow".	To collect evidences/documentation on organization models and work flows for the specific CR in the clinical application
"Teaching for the insiders".	To analyse the training paths for the insiders, considering the different roles
"Regulatory framework (including cybersecurity) and ethical aspects"	To collect evidences/documentation on the regulatory framework (including also the cybersecurity) and ethical issues with reference to the two detected macro areas

References

1. Dolic, Z.; Castro, R.; Moarcas, A. Robots in Healthcare: A Solution or a Problem? Study for the Committee on Environment, Public Health, and Food Safety. Luxembourg: Policy Department for Economic, Scientific and Quality of Life Policies, European Parliament. 2019. Available online: https://www.europarl.europa.eu/RegData/etudes/IDAN/2019/638391/IPOL_IDA(2019)638391_EN.pdf (accessed on 20 November 2021).
2. Available online: https://www.granta-automation.co.uk/news/advantages-and-disadvantages-of-robotic-automation/ (accessed on 20 November 2021).
3. Available online: https://www.futurelearn.com/info/courses/begin-robotics/0/steps/2845 (accessed on 20 November 2021).
4. Available online: https://www.delveinsight.com/blog/robotics-in-healthcare (accessed on 20 November 2021).
5. Stahl, B.C.; Coeckelbergh, M. Ethics of healthcare robotics: Towards responsible research and innovation. *Robot. Auton. Syst.* **2016**, *86*, 152–161. [CrossRef]
6. Gordon, J.-S. Building Moral Robots: Ethical Pitfalls and Challenges. *Sci. Eng. Ethic* **2020**, *26*, 141–157. [CrossRef] [PubMed]
7. Available online: https://pubmed.ncbi.nlm.nih.gov/?term=robot%5BTitle%2FAbstract%5D&sort=date (accessed on 8 September 2021).
8. Fosch-Villaronga, E.; Mahler, T. Cybersecurity, safety and robots: Strengthening the link between cybersecurity and safety in the context of care robots. *Comput. Law Secur. Rev.* **2021**, *41*, 105528. [CrossRef]
9. Yaacoub, J.-P.A.; Noura, H.N.; Salman, O.; Chehab, A. Robotics cyber security: Vulnerabilities, attacks, countermeasures, and recommendations. *Int. J. Inf. Secur.* **2021**, 1–44. [CrossRef]
10. Available online: http://www.rssp.salute.gov.it/rssp2012/paginaCapitoloRssp2012.jsp?sezione=ssn&capitolo=modelli&lingua=italiano (accessed on 8 September 2021).

11. Cochrane, A.L. *Effectiveness and Efficiency: Random Reflections on Health Services*; Nuffield Provincial Hospital Trust: London, UK, 1972.
12. Sackett, D.L.; Rosenberg, W.M.; Gray, J.M.; Haynes, R.B.; Richardson, W.S. Evidence-based medicine: What it is and what it isn't. *Br. Med. J.* **1996**, *312*, 71–72. [CrossRef]
13. Haynes, R.B.; Sackett, D.L. Richardson W. Evidence-based medicine: How to practice & teach EBM. *Can. Med. Assoc. J.* **1997**, *157*, 788.
14. Available online: https://www.ebm-guidelines.com/dtk/ebmg/home (accessed on 20 November 2021).
15. Luce, B.R.; Drummond, M.; Jönsson, B.; Neumann, P.J.; Schwartz, J.S.; Siebert, U.; Sullivan, S.D. EBM, HTA, and CER: Clearing the Confusion. *Milbank Q.* **2010**, *88*, 256–276. [CrossRef]
16. Office of Technology Assessment. 1978. Assessing the Efficacy and Safety of Medical Technologies. September. NTIS order #PB-286929. Available online: http://www.fas.org/ota/reports/7805.pdf (accessed on 25 November 2009).
17. INAHTA (International Network of Agencies for Health Technology Assessment). 2009. HTA Resources. Available online: http://www.inahta.org/HTA/ (accessed on 25 November 2009).
18. Candiani, G.; Colombo, C.; Draghini, R.; Magrini, M.; Mosconi, P.; Nonino, F.; Satolli, R. *Come Organizzare Una Conferenza di Consenso*; Manuale Metodologico; ISS-SNLG: Roma, Italy, 2009.
19. Arcelloni, M.C.; Broggi, F.; Cortese, S.; Della Corte, G.; Pirozzolo, V. CONSENSUS CONFERENCE: UNO STRUMENTO PER LA PRATICA CLINICA Riferimenti storico-metodologici e stato dell'arte dei lavori italiani sul Disturbo Primario del Linguaggio e sui Disturbi Specifici dell'Apprendimento. Available online: https://rivistedigitali.erickson.it/il-tnpee/archivio/vol-1-n-1/riferimenti-storico-metodologici-e-stato-dellarte-dei-lavori-italiani-sul-disturbo-primario-del-linguaggio-e-sui-disturbi-specifici-dellapprendimento/ (accessed on 20 November 2021).
20. McGlynn, E.A.; Kosecoff, J.; Brook, R.H. Format and Conduct of Consensus Development Conferences. *Int. J. Technol. Assess. Heal. Care* **1990**, *6*, 450–469. [CrossRef]
21. Agence Nationale d'Accréditation et d'Évaluation en Santé; Les Conférences de consensus. *Base Méthodologique Pour Leur Réalisation en France*; ANAES: Paris, France, 1999.
22. Available online: https://pubmed.ncbi.nlm.nih.gov/?term=%28consensus+conference%29+AND+%28robot%5BTitle%2FAbstract%5D%29&sort=date (accessed on 20 November 2021).
23. Gimigliano, F.; Palomba, A.; Arienti, C.; Morone, G.; Perrero, L.; Agostini, M.; Aprile, I.; Paci, M.; Casanova, E.; Marino, D.; et al. Robot-assisted arm therapy inneurological health conditions: Rationale and methodology for the evidencesynthesis in the CICERONE Italian Consensus Conference. *Eur. J. Phys. Rehabil. Med.* **2021**, *57*, 824–830. [CrossRef]
24. Calabrò, R.S.; Sorrentino, G.; Cassio, A.; Mazzoli, D.; Andrenelli, E.; Bizzarini, E.; Campanini, I.; Carmignano, S.M.; Cerulli, S.; Chisari, C.; et al. Robotic-assisted gait rehabilitation following stroke: A systematic review of current guidelines and practical clinical recommendations. *Eur. J. Phys. Rehabil. Med.* **2021**, *57*, 460–471. [CrossRef]
25. Morone, G.; Palomba, A.; Martino Cinnera, A.; Agostini, M.; Aprile, I.; Arienti, C.; Paci, M.; Casanova, E.; Marino, D.; LARosa, G.; et al. "CICERONE" Italian Consensus Conference on Robotic in Neurorehabilitation.Systematic review of guidelines to identify recommendations for upper limb robotic rehabilitation after stroke. *Eur. J. Phys. Rehabil. Med.* **2021**, *57*, 238–245. [CrossRef]
26. Rossi, S.; Antal, A.; Bestmann, S.; Bikson, M.; Brewer, C.; Brockmöller, J.; Carpenter, L.L.; Cincotta, M.; Chen, R.; Daskalakis, J.D.; et al. Basis of this article began with a Consensus Statement from the IFCN Workshop on "Present, Future of TMS: Safety, Ethical Guidelines", Siena, October 17–20, 2018, updating through April 2020. Safety and recommendations for TMS use in healthy subjects and patient populations, with updates on training, ethical and regulatory issues: Expert Guidelines. *Clin. Neurophysiol.* **2021**, *132*, 269–306. [CrossRef] [PubMed]
27. Morone, G.; Cocchi, I.; Paolucci, S.; Iosa, M. Robot-assisted therapy for arm recovery for stroke patients: State of the art and clinical implication. *Expert Rev. Med. Devices* **2020**, *17*, 223–233. [CrossRef] [PubMed]
28. Vanlander, A.E.; Mazzone, E.; Collins, J.W.; Mottrie, A.M.; Rogiers, X.M.; van der Poel, H.G.; Van Herzeele, I.; Satava, R.M.; Gallagher, A.G. Orsi Consensus Meeting on European Robotic Training (OCERT): Results from the First Multispecialty Consensus Meeting on Training in Robot-assisted Surgery. *Eur. Urol.* **2020**, *78*, 713–716. [CrossRef]
29. Collins, J.W.; Levy, J.; Stefanidis, D.; Gallagher, A.; Coleman, M.; Cecil, T.; Ericsson, A.; Mottrie, A.; Wiklund, P.; Ahmed, K.; et al. Utilising the Delphi Process to Develop a Proficiency-based Progression Train-the-trainer Course for Robotic Surgery Training. *Eur. Urol.* **2019**, *75*, 775–785. [CrossRef]
30. Cheung, T.T.; Han, H.S.; She, W.H.; Chen, K.H.; Chow, P.K.H.; Yoong, B.K.; Lee, K.F.; Kubo, S.; Tang, C.N.; Wakabayashi, G. The Asia Pacific Consensus Statement on Laparoscopic Liver Resection for Hepatocellular Carcinoma: A Report from the 7th Asia-Pacific Primary Liver Cancer Expert Meeting Held in Hong Kong. *Liver Cancer* **2018**, *7*, 28–39. [CrossRef] [PubMed]
31. Montagnini, A.L.; Røsok, B.I.; Asbun, H.J.; Barkun, J.; Besselink, M.G.; Boggi, U.; Conlon, K.C.; Fingerhut, A.; Han, H.S.; Hansen, P.D.; et al. Standardizing terminology for minimally invasive pancreatic resection. *HPB* **2017**, *19*, 182–189. [CrossRef]
32. Collins, J.W.; Patel, H.; Adding, C.; Annerstedt, M.; Dasgupta, P.; Khan, S.M.; Artibani, W.; Gaston, R.; Piechaud, T.; Catto, J.W.; et al. Enhanced Recovery After Robot-assisted Radical Cystectomy: EAU Robotic Urology Section Scientific Working Group Consensus View. *Eur. Urol.* **2016**, *70*, 649–660. [CrossRef]
33. Chan, K.G.; Guru, K.; Wiklund, P.; Catto, J.; Yuh, B.; Novara, G.; Murphy, D.G.; Al-Tartir, T.; Collins, J.W.; Zhumkhawala, A.; et al. Pasadena Consensus Panel. Robot- assisted radical cystectomy and urinary diversion: Technical recommendations from the Pasadena Consensus Panel. *Eur. Urol.* **2015**, *3*, 423–431. [CrossRef]

34. Wilson, T.G.; Guru, K.; Rosen, R.C.; Wiklund, P.; Annerstedt, M.; Bochner, B.H.; Chan, K.G.; Montorsi, F.; Mottrie, A.; Murphy, D.; et al. Best practices in robot-assisted radical cystectomy and urinary reconstruction: Recommendations of the Pasadena Consensus Panel. *Eur. Urol.* **2015**, *67*, 363–375. [CrossRef]
35. Ficarra, V.; Wiklund, P.N.; Rochat, C.H.; Dasgupta, P.; Challacombe, B.J.; Sooriakumaran, P.; Siemer, S.; Suardi, N.; Novara, G.; Mottrie, A. The European Association of Urology Robotic Urology Section (ERUS) survey of robot-assisted radical prostatectomy (RARP). *BJU Int.* **2013**, *111*, 596–603. [CrossRef] [PubMed]
36. Montorsi, F.; Wilson, T.G.; Rosen, R.C.; Ahlering, T.E.; Artibani, W.; Carroll, P.R.; Costello, A.; Eastham, J.A.; Ficarra, V.; Guazzoni, G.; et al. Best practices in robot-assisted radical prostatectomy: Recommendations of the Pasadena Consensus Panel. *Eur. Urol.* **2012**, *62*, 368–381. [CrossRef] [PubMed]
37. Pelton, T.; van Vliet, P.; Hollands, K. Interventions for improving coordination of reach to grasp following stroke: A systematic review. *JBI Libr. Syst. Rev.* **2011**, *9*, 1226–1270. [CrossRef] [PubMed]
38. Wexner, S.D.; Bergamaschi, R.; Lacy, A.; Udo, J.; Brölmann, H.; Kennedy, R.H.; John, H. The current status of robotic pelvic surgery: Results of a multinational interdisciplinary consensus conference. *Surg Endosc.* **2009**, *23*, 438–443. [CrossRef]
39. Kaji, A.H.; Bair, A.; Okuda, Y.; Kobayashi, L.; Khare, R.; Vozenilek, J. Defining systems expertise: Effective simulation at the organizational level–implications for patient safety, disaster surge capacity, and facilitating the systems interface. *Acad. Emerg. Med.* **2008**, *15*, 1098–1103. [CrossRef]
40. Available online: https://pubmed.ncbi.nlm.nih.gov/?term=consensus+conference&sort=date&size=200 (accessed on 20 November 2021).
41. Available online: https://pubmed.ncbi.nlm.nih.gov/?term=%28consensus+conference%29+AND+%28surgery%5BTitle%2FAbstract%5D%29&sort=date (accessed on 20 November 2021).
42. Available online: https://pubmed.ncbi.nlm.nih.gov/?term=%28consensus+conference%29+AND+%28rehabilitation%5BTitle%2FAbstract%5D%29&sort=date&size=200 (accessed on 20 November 2021).
43. Available online: https://pubmed.ncbi.nlm.nih.gov/?term=%28consensus+conference%29+AND+%28assistance%5BTitle%2FAbstract%5D%29&sort=date&size=200 (accessed on 20 November 2021).
44. Available online: https://pubmed.ncbi.nlm.nih.gov/?term=%28consensus+conference%29+AND+%28training+%5BTitle%2FAbstract%5D%29&sort=date&size=200 (accessed on 20 November 2021).
45. Available online: https://www.simfer.it/conferenza-di-consenso-sulla-robotica-23-e-28-ottobre-2020/ (accessed on 20 November 2021).
46. Available online: https://www.iss.it/news/-/asset_publisher/gJ3hFqMQsykM/content/riabilitazione-assistita-da-robot-all-iss-la-consensus-conference (accessed on 20 November 2021).
47. Available online: https://springerhealthcare.it/mr/archivio/la-conferenza-italiana-di-consenso-sulla-robotica-in-riabilitazione/ (accessed on 20 November 2021).
48. Available online: https://www.atia.org/home/at-resources/what-is-at/ (accessed on 20 November 2021).
49. Available online: https://www.who.int/health-topics/assistive-technology#tab=tab_1 (accessed on 20 November 2021).
50. Available online: https://fli.it/tag/consensus-conference/ (accessed on 20 November 2021).
51. Available online: https://www.sidin.org/2020/07/consensus-conference-2020-progetto-cad/ (accessed on 20 November 2021).
52. Regulation (EU) 2017/745 of the European Parliament and of the Council of 5 April 2017 on medical devices, amending Directive 2001/83/EC, Regulation (EC) No 178/2002 and Regulation (EC) No 1223/2009 and repealing Council Directives 90/385/EEC and 93/42/EEC.2017. Available online: https://eur-lex.europa.eu/legal-content/EN/TXT/?uri=CELEX%3A32017R0745 (accessed on 20 November 2021).
53. Boldrini, P.; Bonaiuti, D.; Mazzoleni, S.; Posteraro, F. Rehabilitation assisted by robotic and electromechanical devices for people with neurological disabilities: Contributions for the preparation of a national conference in Italy. *Eur. J. Phys. Rehabil. Med.* **2021**, *57*, 458–459. [CrossRef]
54. Available online: https://digital-strategy.ec.europa.eu/en/policies/cybersecurity-act (accessed on 20 November 2021).

MDPI
St. Alban-Anlage 66
4052 Basel
Switzerland
Tel. +41 61 683 77 34
Fax +41 61 302 89 18
www.mdpi.com

Healthcare Editorial Office
E-mail: healthcare@mdpi.com
www.mdpi.com/journal/healthcare

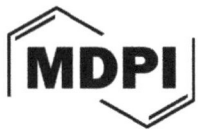

www.ingramcontent.com/pod-product-compliance
Lightning Source LLC
LaVergne TN
LVHW070551100526
838202LV00012B/438